Eggs and Health Promotion

Eggs and Health Promotion

Edited by Ronald Ross Watson

Iowa State Press
A Blackwell Publishing Company

Ronald Ross Watson, Ph.D., is professor in the College of Public Health and School of Medicine, University of Arizona, Tucson. Dr. Watson is a well-recognized nutrition author who has served as editor for more than 50 books on health and nutrition. He is currently a member of several medical organizations including the American Society of Nutritional Sciences, the American College of Nutrition, the American Society of Immunologists, and the American Society for Clinical Investigation. He has conducted nutrition research for 30 years, publishing 450 research articles.

Iowa State Press
2121 State Avenue, Ames, Iowa 50014

Orders: 1-800-862-6657
Office: 1-515-292-0140
Fax: 1-515-292-3348
Web site (secure): www.iowastatepress.com

♾ Printed on acid-free paper in the United States of America

First edition, 2002

Library of Congress Cataloging-in-Publication Data

Eggs and health promotion / editor, Ronald Ross Watson.—1st ed.
p. cm.
Includes bibliographical references and index.
ISBN 0-8138-2798-1 (alk. paper)
1. Eggs—Health aspects.
[DNLM: 1. Eggs. 2. Nutritive Value. QU 145.5 E29 2002] I. Watson, Ronald R. (Ronald Ross)
QP144.E44 E35 2002
613.2′8—dc21 2001005198

The last digit is the print number: 9 8 7 6 5 4 3 2 1

Contents

Preface, vii

Acknowledgments, ix

Contributors, xi

Section 1. Functional Uses of Eggs

1. Functional Uses of Eggs—An Overview, 3
   W.J. Stadelman and Hubert Schmieder
2. The Role of Eggs in American Diets: Health Implications and Benefits, 9
   Jean M. Kerver, Yikyung Park, Won O. Song
3. Designer Eggs: Nutritional and Functional Significance, 19
   Jeong S. Sim and Hoon H. Sunwoo
4. Specialty Eggs: n-3 Fatty Acid–Enriched Eggs, 37
   Elizabeth H. Sheppard
5. Vitamin E Enrichment of Chicken Eggs, 45
   Zeina Makhoul
6. Reducing Infection in Infants with Egg Phospholipids 55
   Yingying Liu and Ronald Ross Watson
7. Generation of Polyclonal Antibodies in the Egg Yolk, 61
   Max Gassmann

Section 2. Cholesterol and Health: Role of Eggs

8. Eggs, Plasma Cholesterol, and Heart Disease Risk, 71
   Donald J. McNamara
9. Eggs and Health: Myths and Misconceptions, 83
   Simin Bolourchi Vaghefi

10. Effect of Dietary Eggs on Human Serum Cholesterol and Coronary Heart Disease, 101
Yinhong Chen and Ronald Ross Watson

11. Eggs and Saturated Fats: Role in Atherosclerosis as Shown by Animal Models, 111
Thomas A. Wilson and Robert J. Nicolosi

12. Health Effects of Docosahexanoic Acid (DHA)–Enriched Eggs, 123
Jin Zhang and Ronald Ross Watson

13. The Correlation between Cholesterol Oxidation Products and Eggs, 133
Jennifer J. Ravia and Ronald Ross Watson

Section 3. Eggs and Disease: Health Promotion

14. Whole Eggs: The Magic Bullet? 141
H.L. "Sam" Queen

15. Enriched Eggs for Human Consumption and the Feeding Pattern of Layers, 155
Carola García, Sergio Cornejo, and Cecilia Albala

16. Predictability of Respiratory Atopy from Egg Hypersensitivity in Children, 171
Kelly Blackstock

17. Effects of Cooking and Storage on the Nutritional Value of Eggs, 177
Giorgio Bedogni and Nino Carlo Battistini

18. The Potential Use of Eggs for the Protein Requirements of Endurance Exercise, 185
Jaclyn Maurer

Index, 193

Preface

For millennia humans have used eggs as key parts of their diets. As the incubation materials for new birds, they contain a great variety of nutrients and materials needed to sustain both life and growth. Recent work suggests that birds may be descended from dinosaurs, meaning that eggs have promoted life for millions of years. The role of eggs as natural sources of vitamins, proteins, fats, and other nutrients is well-known, so this book reviews the myths and misconceptions about eggs. It discusses the fats and lipids in eggs, the nutrients in eggs, eggs' role in health promotion, and the lack of significant risks of eating eggs. The role of eggs in American diets and health is defined. A major focus is on the roles of cholesterol, oxidized lipids, and fats in health promotion. These range from new evidence that eggs have little effect on heart disease to their use in infant food to reduce disease. New research is examined about enhancing lipids in eggs, including vitamin E, to promote human health. A variety of other lipids and fats in eggs are investigated for benefits to health.

Eggs contain fats and cholesterol, important components of cells and needed for life. Some groups have associated high serum levels of these materials with risk of heart disease, while others have linked increased incidence of premature death with low levels. This has led to questions about the benefits of eggs as a food and nutrient source. This controversy is the subject of several chapters in this book. A key hypothesis chapter describes the use of eggs in health promotion and disease prevention.

Recent research shows that eggs often contribute to health by providing essential fatty acids and lipids in cell membranes while contributing little to serum lipids and the risk of heart disease. This book contains some medical hypotheses articles covering such potential roles as eggs as protein sources to build strength in athletes. The general aim of these chapters is to provide up-to-date research on the role of eggs in the health of Americans—for example, how egg consumption benefits women, infants, and the elderly.

A major theme is the use of eggs, with modified nutrient levels and constituents, as an easy and effective method for improving human nutrition. Some authors review the use of eggs from specially fed chickens to provide nutrients to prevent and treat some diseases. Eggs are a mechanism to introduce high levels of carotenoids to Americans, who traditionally eat only 30 percent of the recommended intake. Eggs are also being tested for transporting human immune products into people in a safe and painless manner.

Acknowledgments

Breeding improved hens for better egg production has been scientifically promoted by H.B. Wallace and Hy-line International for more than 63 years. Such programs and companies stimulated this book and its reviews of eggs in health. The encouragement and support of Mr. H. B. Wallace and Wallace Research Inc. was vital to the book's conception and publication. Mr. H.B. Wallace and the Wallace Research Foundation have encouraged studies of the role of nutrition in health in Dr. Watson's laboratory for 22 years. Such research has led to the compilation of recent advances by experts, yielding a dozen books edited by Ronald Ross Watson. He greatly appreciates this stimulation and support, including funding for the editing and preparation of this book. Appreciation is also expressed to Bethany Stevens for her work as an office assistant in getting the manuscripts together.

Contributors

Cecilia Albala, MS
University of Chile
Santa Rosa 11 735
Santiago
Chile

Nino Carlo Battistini, MD
Human Nutrition Chair
Department of Biomedical Sciences
Faculty of Medicine and Surgery
University of Modena and Reggio Emilia
Via Campi 287
41100 Modena
Italy

Giorgio Bedogni, MD
Department of Biomedical Sciences
Faculty of Medicine and Surgery
University of Modena and Reggio Emilia
Via Campi 287
41100 Modena
Italy

Kelly Blackstock, MS, RD
Physiology Department
Gittings 3E
University of Arizona
Tucson, AZ 85724

Yinhong Chen, PhD
College of Pubic Health
University of Arizona
Tucson, AZ 85724

Sergio Cornejo, MS, DVM
Department of Animal Science
Faculty of Veterinary Medicine
University of Chile
Santa Rosa 11 735
Santiago
Chile

Carola García, MSc
Agronomist
Public Health Area
Institute of Nutrition and Food Technology
University of Chile
Macul 5540
Santiago
Chile

Max Gassmann, DVM
Institutes of Physiology and Veterinary Physiology
University of Zürich
CH-8057 Zürich
Switzerland

Jean M. Kerver, MS, RD
Food and Nutrition Database Research Center
Department of Food Science and Human Nutrition
Michigan State University
East Lansing, MI 48824

Yingying Liu, BS, MS
College of Public Health
University of Arizona
Tucson, AZ 85721

Zeina Makhoul, MS, RD
Teaching Assistant
Department of Nutritional Sciences
University of Arizona
Tucson, AZ 85724

Jaclyn Maurer, MS, RD
Research Assistant
Nutritional Assessment Lab
University of Arizona
Tucson, AZ 85721

Donald J. McNamara, PhD
Egg Nutrition Center
1050 17th St. NW, Suite 560
Washington, DC 20036

Robert J. Nicolosi, PhD
Department of Health and Clinical Sciences
Center for Chronic Disease Control and Prevention
University of Massachusetts
Lowell, MA 01854

Yikyung Park, MS
Food and Nutrition Database Research Center
Department of Food Science and Human Nutrition
Michigan State University
East Lansing, MI 48824

H.L. "Sam" Queen, MA, CNS
Author, *Health Realities Journal*
Founder and Director of Research and Development
Institute for Health Realities
5245 Centennial Blvd., Suite 100
Colorado, CO 80919

Jennifer J. Ravia, MS, RD
University of Arizona
Department of Nutrition
Tucson, Arizona 85724

Hubert Schmieder
Chef Emeritus
RHITM Department
Purdue University
West Lafayette, IN 47907

Elizabeth H. Sheppard, MS, RD
3825 N Calle Perdiz
Tucson, AZ 85718

Jeong S. Sim, PhD
Professor, Poultry Nutrition and Product Technology (Chair)
President and CEO, Ovo-biotechnica, Inc., and Designer Food Concept, Inc.
Department of Agricultural, Food and Nutritional Science
University of Alberta
Edmonton, Alberta T6G
Canada

Won O. Song, PhD, MPH, RD
Professor and Associate Dean
Food and Nutrition Database Research Center
Department of Food Science and Human Nutrition
Michigan State University
East Lansing, MI 48824

Dr. W.J. Stadelman, PhD
Professor Emeritus
Food Science Department
Purdue University
West Lafayette, IN 47907

Hoon. H. Sunwoo, PhD
Department of Agricultural, Food, and Nutritional Science
University of Alberta
Edmonton, Alberta T6G 2P5
Canada

Simin Bolourchi Vaghefi, PhD
Associate Professor of Nutrition
College of Health
Nutrition Program
University of North Florida
Jacksonville, FL 32224

Ronald Ross Watson, PhD
College of Pubic Health and School of Medicine
Health Promotion Science Division
1501 N Campbell Ave.
PO Box 245155
University of Arizona
Tucson, AZ 85724

Thomas A. Wilson, PhD, MPH
Department of Health and Clinical Sciences
Center for Chronic Disease Control and Prevention
University of Massachusetts
Lowell, MA 01854

Jin Zhang, PhD
College of Public Health
Health Promotion Science Program
1501 N Campbell Ave.
University of Arizona
PO Box 245155
Tucson, AZ 85724

Section 1

Functional Uses of Eggs

1

Functional Uses of Eggs—An Overview

W.J. Stadelman
and Hubert Schmieder

Introduction

Eggs are a multifunctional food. Egg components have the ability to coagulate when heated, to act as emulsifiers in oil and water formulations, and to form foams when whipped. Components of the egg make it an excellent source of high-quality protein, vitamins, and trace minerals. Eggs are used in some candies and icings to enhance color and flavor while minimizing crystal formation. A book published in 1977 lists 979 methods of preparing various egg dishes.[1]

Some nonfood uses of eggs include their use as a source of avidin and lysozyme, as well as for fining, softening, and polishing red wines. The egg can also be used as a carrier of antibodies against some diseases of humans and animals.

Eggs are composed of four distinct and separable parts: shell, shell membranes, albumen, and yolk. Each of these parts has value for different applications. Shell eggs are frequently converted into egg products such as liquid, frozen, or dehydrated whole eggs, albumen, yolk, as well as blends.

Nutritional Value

The nutritional value of the egg is extensively discussed in the following chapters. The egg is the perfect food for a chick; however, it is deficient in vitamin C for humans. The portion of the egg normally eaten is also deficient in calcium. Most of the calcium in an egg is found in the shell as calcium carbonate. The exact quantity of various fatty acids, minerals, and vitamins is dependent on the level of each in the diet of the hen. Levels of most nutrients in the egg are influenced by age, breed or strain, season of the year, and diet of the hen.[2] While most of the variations are relatively slight, the fatty acid composition can be markedly modified by changes in the fatty acid composition of the hen's diet. The vitamin and trace mineral content are also variable depending on the amounts of the particular compound in the diet of the hen.

Although the shell of the egg is not generally considered edible, finely powdered eggshell can be utilized as a calcium source for humans.[3] The absorption of eggshell calcium is greater than for conventional calcium sources. Finely ground eggshell is used as a calcium enrichment in some breads and confections.

Coagulation

Coagulation is the phenomenon of a liquid changing to a semisolid or solid. Heat coagulation can occur in both egg white and egg yolk. The proteins of the egg white coagulate at various temperatures. Conalbumin or ovotransferrin coagulates at 57.3°C; lysozyme at 81.5°C.[4] The other proteins of the albumen coagulate at intermediate temperatures between these extremes. Egg yolk begins to coagulate at 65°C and ceases to flow at 70°C. The action of coagulation is an unfolding of protein coils when heated and a bonding between the molecules that results in a change from a transparent watery liquid into an opaque, polycondensated solid in the irreversible reaction.[5] The success of many cooked foods is dependent on the heat coagulation of egg proteins.

The effects of heat coagulation are most evident in the preparation of hard-cooked or fried eggs. The firmness of the coagulated albumen is directly related to the time and temperature of heat application. Eggs are frequently included as an ingredient in meatloaf to bind the other ingredients together, a result of coagulation of the egg proteins. Eggs are included in quiches, custards, flans, crepes, and many other foods for this binding action of the heated proteins. Eggs are included in batter mixtures to coat various foods prior to deep fat frying. The egg proteins bind the batter to the surface of the food product. The coagulation property of egg proteins is used also in clarification of clear consommé. The albumen of one egg is added to each 5 quarts of cold white consommé, which is then heated to coagulate the egg proteins. The particulate materials are collected in the white consommé, and the broth is then strained through cheesecloth to remove the egg white and particulates.[6]

Foaming

A foam is a colloidal dispersion in which a gaseous phase is dispersed in a liquid or solid phase.[4] The mechanism of foam formation during whipping of liquid egg products is described as an unfolding of the protein molecules so that the polypeptide chains exist with the long axes parallel to the surface.[7] This change in molecular configuration results in a loss of solubility or precipitation of some of the albumen, which collects at the liquid-air interface. Many foods are capable of foaming; eggs are especially effective in this capacity. For a foam to be of value in cookery, it must be relatively stable. Egg foaming is brought about by whipping of the liquid egg products. Whole eggs can be used to produce foam for yellow sponge cakes. However, egg whites are generally used for getting maximum foams. Egg whites with a large percentage of thick white take longer to whip to maximum foam volume, but the foam formed is more stable than foams formed from lower-quality eggs that contain a higher percentage of thin white. Chefs have claimed for years that whipping of egg white in a copper bowl yields superior products. In a test at a cooking school,[8] no difference was found in foam volume. However, when the foamed product was baked, the end product had a significant increase in volume. It was postulated that the conalbumin of the egg white complexed with the copper, forming a product with a lowered heat sensitivity. This allowed the air bubbles in the product to expand farther before being set due to coagulation of the proteins.

Eggs are used for their foaming ability in the preparation of meringues, angel food cakes, sponge cakes, and mousses.

Emulsification

The reduction of interfacial tension between water and oil is the first step in the formation of an emulsion.[9] The surface active agents in egg yolk are essential to its function in emulsification. The surface active agents form a film around the oil globules and prevent their coalescence in emulsion food products. Egg yolk is itself an emulsion. The emulsifying capacity of egg yolk is not altered by modifying the fatty acid composition of the yolk.[10] In cookery, the emulsifying function of the egg yolk is utilized in the preparation of hollandaise and other sauces. In food manufacture, this function is used in the production of mayonnaise and salad dressings.

Color

The naturally occurring pigments in chicken egg yolk include the alcohol-soluble xanthophylls, lutein, and zeaxanthin. The color of the yolk is influenced by the concentration of these pigments in the ration of the hen. It is possible to produce various yolk colors by feeding the hen fat-soluble dyes. Egg yolk color is of importance in the manufacture of noodles, sponge cakes, and scrambled eggs. In the hard cooking of eggs, a greenish color is formed on the surface of the yolk of an overcooked egg due to the formation of ferrous sulfide produced at the interface of the yolk and the albumen.[11]

Flavor

Fresh eggs have a very mild flavor. Eggs will absorb off-flavors if stored with apples, petroleum products, odoriferous vegetables, or other sources of odors. With long-term storage eggs will develop a stale flavor.

Fresh egg flavor is desirable in scrambled eggs, fried eggs, poached eggs, soft-cooked eggs, and eggnog. As egg flavor is mild it blends well with the flavor of all foods.

Inhibition of Crystal Formation

The ability of egg whites to minimize crystallization of sugars in icings and candies has been known for many years.[12] In candy manufacture egg white is used to help ensure creamy smoothness as well as whiteness in such confections as divinity fudge and fondant. As the hot syrup is added to the beaten egg white, the albumen forms thin films around the tiny sugar crystals and prevents them from clustering together, which results in a grainy and crumbly candy.

Nonfood Uses

The principal nonfood use of the egg is to reproduce the species. With the great increase in the consumption of poultry meat, the number of eggs required for chick production has expanded greatly. Several other nonfood uses of eggs were summarized by USDA personnel.[13]

Industrial egg albumen is used in finishing certain types of leather, particularly glazed, colored stock. Inedible eggs are utilized also in animal feedstuffs and plant fertilizers. Eggs are often fed to show animals, such as dogs and horses, to improve the glossy sheen of the fur coat.

Another important use of eggs is the production of vaccines in chick embryos. Vaccines for many infectious diseases are now produced in quantity using the chick embryo. These vaccines include several pox diseases, lymphogranuloma, and influenza of humans; for many diseases of the fowl; as well as vesicular stomatitis and infectious encephalomyelitis for horses.

The use of laying hens for the production of antibodies in the hen that are transferred to the egg is discussed in chapter 12. Currently research is underway to adapt the antibody therapy in the treatment of the HIV virus responsible for acquired immune deficiency syndrome (AIDS).[14] Although the virus cannot be eradicated, daily consumption of IgY from eggs of hens properly infected with the HIV virus can control the negative effects of reduced immunity to opportunistic infections to some extent.

A quite different use of eggs is in artistic and cultural applications.[15] The decoration of eggs for Easter is an international activity. Eggshells were decorated for King Edward I of England, who presented the gold-leafed eggs to his court as gifts in the 13th century. During the 16th century, in France, Louis XV presented Madame Du Barry the gift of a gilded egg containing the "surprise" of a cupid. Shell egg decoration reached its zenith in Russia when Peter Carl Fabergé (1846–1920) decorated eggs for the czars.

Fragments of eggshell have been used in the preparation of mosaics dating back to the 15th century. Tempera painting uses an emulsion of egg yolk thinned with water. It dries quickly and is very stable. Eggs have been used in myths of creation, witchcraft and magic, fertility, purity, and resurrection.[16] As such, the egg has been used as a symbol for the cosmos, as a charm to encourage reproduction, as a medium for the exorcism of devils, and as a symbol of rebirth and has been called the devil's food. The egg has often been revered as a symbol of life; some early societies even prohibited the use of eggs as food.

Eggshell membranes are generally considered a waste. However, studies in Japan have shown that protein products prepared from hydrolyzed egg membrane are beneficial in stimulating skin regeneration after injury. Egg membrane protein tends to allow growth of human skin fibroblasts and facilitates the production of type III collagen. The egg membrane protein is currently being used for its emollient properties in many cosmetics and toiletries.[3]

Egg white is used in the clarification of red table wines. In a process known as "fining," egg white is mixed with 0.5 to 0.9 percent salt water (60 ml albumen to 40 ml water) to solubilize the globulins in the egg white. The diluted egg white is then beaten to a froth and mixed with about 10 volumes of wine before being added to the main volume of wine.[17,18] The albumen from one to two eggs is used for a barrel of wine (225 l). The solution is added to the wine and mixed well. The egg albumen interacts with the higher polymeric phenols and tannins to soften and polish the red wines.

From this brief review, it is apparent that all parts of the egg have been found to have value either as food or for other purposes. More details on the major functions of the egg can be found in Yang and Baldwin.[4]

References

1. Bickel, W. Hering's Dictionary of Classical and Modern Cookery. 5th ed. London: Virtue and Company, 1997, p. 118.
2. Stadelman, W.J., and Pratt, D.E. Factors influencing composition of the hen's egg. World's Poult Sci J 1989;45:247.
3. Sugura, N., Horiike, S., Masida, Y., Kunou, M., and Kokubu, T. Bioavailability and commercial use of eggshell calcium, membrane proteins and yolk lecithin products. In Egg Nutrition and Biotechnology, Sim, J.S., Nakai, S., and Guenter, W., eds. New York: CABI Publishing, 1999, chap. 17.
4. Yang, Sheng-Chin, and Baldwin, R.E. Functional properties of eggs in foods. In Egg Science and Technology, 4th ed., Stadelman, W.J., and Cotterill, O.J., eds. Binghamton, NY: Haworth Press, 1995, chap. 16.
5. Coenders, A. The Chemistry of Cooking. Park Ridge, NJ: Parthenon Publishing Co., 1992, p. 119.
6. Escoffier, A. The Escoffier Cook Book. New York: Crown Publishers, 1969, p. 4.
7. Griswold, R.M. The Experimental Study of Foods. Boston, MA: Houghton Mifflin Co., 1962.
8. Corriher, S.O. Cookwise, the Hows and Whys of Successful Cooking. New York: William Morrow and Co., 1997, p. 234.
9. Vincent, R., Powrie, W.D., and Fennema, O. Surface activity of yolk, plasma and dispersions of yolk fractions. J Food Sci 1966;31:643.
10. Pankey, R.D., and Stadelman, W.J. Effect of dietary fats on some chemical and functional properties of eggs. J Food Sci 1969;34:312.
11. Baker, R.L., Darfler, J., and Lifshitz, A. Factors affecting the discoloration of hard cooked egg yolks. Poult Sci 1967;46:664.
12. Swanson, E.L. Egg whites and sugar crystals. US Egg Poult Mag 1933;39(9):32.
13. USDA. Eggs and egg products. U.S. Dep Agric Circ 583, 1941.
14. Coleman, M. Using egg antibodies to treat diseases. In Egg Nutrition and Biotechnology, Sim, J.S., Nakai, S., and Guenter, W., eds. New York: CABI Publishing, 2000, p. 351.
15. Galyean, R.D., and Cotterill, O.J. Nonfood uses of eggs. In Egg Science and Technology, 4th ed., Stadelman, W.J., and Cotterill, O.J., eds. Binghamton, NY: Haworth Press, 1995, chap. 20.
16. Newall, V. An Egg at Easter. Bloomington: Indiana Univ. Press, 1971.

17. Amerine, M.A., Berg, H.W., Kunkee, R.E. Ough, C.S., Singleton, V.L., and Webb, A.D. The Technology of Wine Making, 4th ed. Westport, CN: AVI Publishing Co., 1982, p. 317.
18. Margalit, Yair. Concepts in Wine Chemistry, South San Francisco, CA: Wine Appreciation Guild Ltd., 1997, p. 287.

2

The Role of Eggs in American Diets: Health Implications and Benefits

Jean M. Kerver,
Yikyung Park,
and Won O. Song

INTRODUCTION

Over the years, the American public has been advised to decrease its consumption of eggs. Americans have responded to this message by decreasing per capita egg consumption from 402 eggs per year in 1945 to 236 eggs per year in 1995.[19] This dietary recommendation is based on the cholesterol content of eggs, even though dietary cholesterol has been shown to be only a minor contributor to elevated serum cholesterol concentrations.[19]

In a study examining dietary trends of older Americans from 1977 to 1996, egg consumption decreased by 46 percent in males and 29 percent in females.[6] In the same analysis, it was concluded that the elderly should increase their intakes of food energy, dietary fiber, vitamin E, folate, calcium, magnesium, and zinc. As shown in this chapter, as a result of being advised to limit egg use, Americans may be depriving themselves of a significant source of beneficial nutrients.

WAYS TO ASSESS THE ROLE OF EGGS IN THE AMERICAN DIET

The composition of the U.S. diet is primarily evaluated by use of food disappearance or individual food consumption data. Food disappearance data provide an estimate of per capita food availability. These data do not directly measure actual food consumption, but rather, using a balance sheet approach, they estimate the amount of each commodity food that is available for human consumption. Beginning year inventories of total food production and imports are used after subtracting exports, industrial uses, farm inputs, and end-of-year inventories.[17] These data do not take into account food fed to pets and food losses due to spoilage, disposal of inedible parts, and trimming by the consumer. However, they do provide estimates of change in overall patterns of food disappearance over time.

Estimates of individual food and nutrient consumption are also provided by national nutrition surveys, such as the USDA's Continuing Survey of Food Intakes by Individuals (CSFII) and the Center for Disease Control's National Health and Nutrition Examination Surveys (NHANES). These surveys sample the U.S. population and obtain information about recent and usual dietary intake using 24-hour recalls and food frequency questionnaires. The most recent national nutrition survey data available are from the 1994–1996 CSFII and NHANES III (1988–1994). The surveys differ in that the CSFII includes data for 3 consecutive days, and the NHANES III includes physical examinations and serum chemistries in addition to food intake data for one 24-hour period. The results of both studies can be extrapolated to the U.S. population when proper sample weights are applied to the analyses.

Consumption of Eggs in the American Diet

Food supply data have shown that eggs accounted for 9 percent of the total meat equivalent servings in 1996.[13] In the 1989–1991 CSFII, approximately 40 percent of individuals reported egg use on at least 1 of the 3 days of the survey.[17] Egg use was defined as consumption of whole eggs, egg whites, egg yolks, meringues, egg substitutes, baby-food egg yolks, and mixtures having egg as a main ingredient, such as omelets, egg salad, or egg sandwiches, coded as a single item. Eggs that were ingredients in food mixtures coded as a single item and tabulated under another food group (e.g., eggs in baked goods, which were tabulated under grain products) were excluded. Despite the high percentage of people reporting egg use, mean egg intake per person per day was only 17 g. For reference, one large egg weighs 50 g. In addition, egg use varied by race, sex, and age. Higher percentages of black than white males and females 20 years of age and older reported using eggs, including whole eggs, egg substitutes, and eggs in other forms. The highest percentage of adults reporting egg consumption were in the income category 130 percent of poverty. Because eggs and egg substitutes were not listed separately, consumption of each type of product could not be examined in this report.[17]

Nutritive Value of Eggs

The nutrient composition of a large, raw, fresh egg is shown in Table 2.1. As shown, a single egg provides 74.5 kcal energy to the diet, with protein and fat being the primary source of this energy. A single egg contains 212.5 mg cholesterol and 5.01 g of total fat. However, only 1.6 g of total fat is saturated, and more than half is unsaturated (1.9 g monounsaturated and 0.7 g polyunsaturated). The fact that eggs contain significant amounts of other nutrients has been largely ignored.

U.S. food supply data on nutrient content show that significant amounts of energy, protein, total fat, saturated fatty acids (SFAs), monounsaturated fatty acids (MUFAs), polyunsaturated fatty acids (PUFAs), cholesterol, vitamin A, vitamin E, thiamin, riboflavin, vitamin B_6, vitamin B_{12}, folate, iron, calcium, phosphorus, magnesium, potassium, and zinc come from eggs (Table 2.2). No significant amount of carbohydrate, fiber, vitamin C, carotenoids, niacin, sodium, or copper is available from eggs in the U.S. food supply.

Using one 24-hour recall from the 1989–1991 CSFII, Subar et al. reported the dietary sources of nutrients among U.S. adults.[31] Eggs were a notable source of energy, protein, total fat, SFAs, PUFAs, MUFAs, cholesterol, vitamin E, vitamin A, folate, riboflavin, vitamin B_6, vitamin B_{12}, calcium, phosphorus, iron, and zinc (Table 2.3). Eggs were not a notable source of carbohydrates, fiber, vitamin C, carotenoids, thiamin, niacin, sodium, potassium, magnesium, or copper.

In a similar report, Subar et al. described the dietary sources of nutrients in American children.[32] Eggs were found to be a significant source of energy, protein, total fat, SFAs, cholesterol, vitamin E, vitamin A, folate, iron, and zinc (Table 2.4). Eggs were not a notable source of carbohydrate, fiber, vitamin C, carotenoids, calcium, or magnesium. Other nutrients were not reported.

Table 2.1. Nutrient composition of a whole, raw, fresh egg

Nutrient		Units	One large egg (50 g)
Macro nutrients	Energy	kcal	74.50
	Protein	g	6.25
	Total fat	g	5.01
	Carbohydrate	g	0.61
Minerals	Phosphorus	mg	89.00
	Potassium	mg	60.50
	Sodium	mg	63.00
	Calcium	mg	24.50
	Magnesium	mg	5.00
	Iron	mg	0.72
	Zinc	mg	0.55
	Copper	mg	0.01
	Manganese	mg	0.01
	Selenium	mcg	15.40
Vitamins	Vitamin A	IU	317.50
		RE	95.50
	Vitamin D	IU	26.00
	Pantothenic acid	mg	0.63
	Vitamin E	mg α-TE	0.53
	Riboflavin	mg	0.25
	Vitamin B_6	mg	0.07
	Niacin	mg	0.04
	Thiamin	mg	0.03
	Folate	mcg	23.50
	Vitamin B_{12}	mcg	0.50
Lipids	Monounsaturated fatty acids	g	1.91
	Saturated fatty acids	g	1.55
	Polyunsaturated fatty acids	g	0.68
	Cholesterol	mg	212.50

Source: http://www.nal.usda.gov/fnic/cgi-bin/list_nut.pl.

Table 2.2. Nutrients available from eggs in the U.S. food supply

Nutrient	Percentage of total food supply
Cholesterol	33.2
Riboflavin	6.4
Folate	5.1
Vitamin E	4.3
Vitamin A	4.3
Protein	3.9
Vitamin B_{12}	3.7
Phosphorus	3.6
Zinc	2.8
Iron	2.4
Vitamin B_6	2.1
Total fat	2.0
Monounsaturated fatty acids	1.8
Saturated fatty acids	1.7
Calcium	1.7
Polyunsaturated fatty acids	1.4
Energy	1.3
Potassium	1.1
Magnesium	0.9
Thiamin	0.8
Copper	0.3
Carbohydrate	0.1
Niacin	0.1

Source: Reference 18.

Effect of Limiting Egg Consumption on Nutrition

Taken together, results of the aforementioned studies suggest that a diet that excludes eggs will also exclude many beneficial nutrients found in eggs. The hypothesis that Americans may be depriving themselves of a significant source of nutrients by limiting egg consumption was recently tested using NHANES III data.[30] The main purposes of this study were (1) to assess the nutritional significance of eggs in the American diet and (2) to estimate the degree of association between egg consumption and serum cholesterol concentration. To meet these objectives, the following subjects were excluded from the statistical analyses: subjects with unreliable dietary recall records as coded by the National Center for Health Statistics (NCHS), pregnant and lactating women, those taking drugs for hyperlipidemia or unspecified heart disease, or those consuming egg white products. Serum cholesterol data from subjects who reported changing their diet in the past year due to high serum cholesterol levels were not included.

Characteristics of egg consumers were similar to those reported in CSFII. Nearly 20 percent of the population reported consuming eggs in the 24-hour recall. Egg consump-

Table 2.3. Nutrients provided by eggs in diets of American adults (1989–1991 CSFII)

Nutrient	Percentage of dietary total	Ranking[a]
Cholesterol	29.1	1
Riboflavin	5.2	5
Vitamin E	4.7	6
Vitamin A	3.5	8
Vitamin B_{12}	3.5	6
Protein	3.2	7
Phosphorus	2.9	7
Folate	2.8	7
Toal fat	2.7	13
Monounsaturated fatty acids	2.7	14
Saturated fatty acids	2.4	14
Polyunsaturated fatty acids	≈1.0	12
Energy	≈1.0	19
Vitamin B_6	≈1.0	15
Calcium	≈1.0	9
Iron	≈1.0	13
Zinc	≈1.0	10

Source. Reference 31.
[a]Foods were ranked out of all foods contributing at least 1 percent of the nutrient.

Table 2.4. Nutrients provided by eggs in diets of American children (1989–1991 CSFII)

Nutrient	Percentage of dietary total	Ranking[a]
Cholesterol	23.8	1
Vitamin E	3.9	10
Vitamin A	2.8	7
Protein	2.4	7
Folate	1.9	9
Total fat	1.9	16
Saturated fatty acids	1.6	18
Zinc	1.5	14
Iron	1.4	15
Energy	1.1	28

Source. Reference 32.
[a]Foods were ranked out of all foods contributing at least 1percent of the nutrient.

tion was significantly influenced by gender, ethnicity, age, and education level. Egg ingestion was higher in males than females and in Mexican-Americans compared with other ethnic groups. Older Americans and people with lower education levels were more likely to eat eggs than younger or more educated people.

Daily nutrient intake of egg consumers was greater than that of subjects who did not consume eggs for all nutrients studied except dietary fiber and vitamin B_6 ($p < 0.05$). Among egg consumers, eggs contributed <10 percent of energy and vitamin B_6; 10–20 percent of total, saturated, and polyunsaturated fat; 10–20 percent of total folate; and 20–30 percent of vitamins A, E, and B_{12}. In contrast to those subjects who did not consume eggs, a greater percentage of egg consumers had adequate intake (as measured by Estimated Average Requirement [EAR] or ≥70 percent Recommended Daily Allowance [RDA]) of vitamin B_{12}, vitamin A, vitamin E, and vitamin C than inadequate intake (<EAR or <70 percent RDA). Compared with egg consumers, a greater proportion of those subjects who did not consume eggs had inadequate intakes of vitamin B_{12} (10 percent versus 20 percent), vitamin A (16 percent versus 21 percent), vitamin E (14 percent versus 22 percent), and vitamin C (15 percent versus 20 percent).

Relationship between Eggs, Serum Cholesterol, and Coronary Heart Disease

Results of our analysis of NHANES III data refute the hypothesis that egg consumption increases serum cholesterol.[30] After controlling for the effect of demographic (age, gender, and ethnicity) and lifestyle variables (smoking and physical activity), and excluding subjects expected of having high cholesterol levels, we found that (1) dietary cholesterol consumption did not appear to have any significant bearing on the serum cholesterol concentration and (2) total serum cholesterol concentration was negatively related to frequency of egg consumption. Subjects who reported eating four or more eggs per week had significantly lower mean serum cholesterol concentrations than those who reported eating one or fewer eggs per week (193 mg/dl versus 197 mg/dl; $p < 0.01$). The fact that the average serum cholesterol level of subjects was less than 220 mg/dl indicates that we were largely successful in removing individuals with known high cholesterol levels from our analysis.

Our findings support results of recent clinical studies that have shown that egg consumption and serum cholesterol concentrations are not directly related.[5,7,11,34] An epidemiological study involving 37,851 men and 80,082 women revealed that consumption of up to one egg per day does not affect the risk of developing coronary heart disease or stroke.[12] In this study, egg consumption was positively associated with smoking, lower physical activity, and ingestion of a high-fat diet. When these factors were adjusted for in the analysis, egg consumption was not positively associated with risk of coronary heart disease. This suggests that overall eating patterns need to be examined when epidemiological data is used to examine the effect of a single food (such as eggs) on risk of developing diseases.

Utilizing data from the American Heart Association (1998), McNamara showed that there is a negative relationship between per capita egg consumption of men in 24 industrialized countries and coronary vascular disease (CVD) mortality rates.[19] The highest per capita egg-consuming countries (Japan, Mexico, Spain, and France) had the lowest CVD mortality rates of the countries studied. A common feature of diets in these countries is low intake of saturated fat and high intake of fruits and vegetables. In a study by Kushi et al., those with coronary heart disease (CHD) had a lower vegetable-food score (–0.44 versus 0.06) and a higher animal-food score (0.24 versus –0.04) than healthy controls.[15] These data suggest that high intake of saturated fat and low intake of fruits and vegetables are involved in development of CHD. Because saturated fat and cholesterol are highly related covariables, cholesterol intake may simply serve as a marker for high intake of saturated fat and low intake of fruits and vegetables.

As shown in Tables 2.1 to 2.4, eggs are a good source of vitamin E, B vitamins, and folate. Antioxidants and B vitamins have been shown to protect against development of coronary disease in humans.[14,22,24] Folate deficiency is associated with elevated plasma levels of homocysteine, a risk factor for occlusive cardiovascular disease.[24,26,33] Supplementation of diets with folic acid reduces plasma homocysteine concentrations in healthy volunteers and cardiac patients[1,2,16,25,36] and reduces the risk of coronary heart disease.[23] These data suggest that by limiting egg consumption, Americans may be depriving themselves of nutrients that guard against development of heart disease. In addition, the fact that nutrients in eggs such as folate, calcium, iron, lutein, and zeaxanthin have been shown to be protective against a host of other diseases such as birth defects,[4,20,27,28,35] colon cancer,[8–10] brain-related disorders such as depression, reduced cognition, Alzheimer's disease,[3,21] and age-related macular degeneration[19,29] indicates that eliminating eggs from your diet for fear of developing heart disease may be detrimental to your health.

Conclusion

Results of clinical and epidemiological studies have shown that diets high in saturated fat and low in fruits and vegetables are associated with development of heart disease. If the influence of saturated fat intake and unhealthy behaviors is controlled for in analyses, no definitive link between cholesterol intake and heart disease has been found. By being wrongly advised to limit egg consumption, Americans may be depriving themselves of a significant source of nutrients that have been shown to protect against a variety of different diseases.

References

1. Brönstrup, A., Hages, M., Prinz-Langenohl, R., and Pietrzik, K. Effects of folic acid and combinations of folic acid and vitamin B-12 on plasma homocysteine concentrations in healthy, young men. Am J Clin Nutr 1998;68:1104–10.

2. Brouwer, I.A., van Dusseldorp, M., Thomas, C., Duran, M., Hautvast, J., Eskes, T., and Steegers–Theunissen, R. Low-dose folic acid supplementation decreases plasma homocysteine concentrations: a randomized trial. Am J Clin Nutr 1999;69:99–104.
3. Clarke R., Smith, D., Jobst, K.A., Refsum, H., Sutton, L., and Ueland, P.M. Folate, vitamin B_{12}, and serum total homocysteine levels in confirmed Alzheimer disease. Arch Neurol 1998;55:1449–55.
4. Czeizel, A.E., and Dudás, I. Prevention of the first occurrence of neural-tube defects by periconceptional vitamin supplementation. N Engl J Med 1992;327:1832–35.
5. Dawber, T.R., Nickerson, R.J., Brand, F.N., and Pool, J. Eggs, serum cholesterol, and coronary heart disease. Am J Clin Nutr 1982;36:617–25.
6. Gerrior, S.A. Dietary changes in older Americans from 1977 to 1996: implications for dietary quality. Fam Econ Nutr Rev 1999;12:3–14.
7. Ginsberg, H.H., Karnally, W., Siddiqyi, M., Holleran, S., Tall, A.R., Ramsey, S.C., Deckelbaum, R.J., Blaner, W.S., and Ramakrishnan, R. A dose-response study of the effects of dietary cholesterol on fasting and postprandial lipid and lipoprotein metabolism in healthy young men. Arterioscler Thromb 1994;14:576–86.
8. Giovannucci, E., Rimm, E.B., Ascherio, A., Stampfer, M.J., Colditz, G.A., and Willett, W.C. Alcohol, low-methionine-low-folate diets, and risk of colon cancer in men. J Natl Cancer Inst 1995;87:265–73.
9. Giovannucci, E., Stampfer, M.J., Colditz, G.A., Hunter, D.J., Fuchs, C., Rosner, B.A., Speitzer, F.E., and Wilett, W.C. Multivitamin use, folate, and colon cancer in women in the Nurse's Health Study. Ann Intern Med 1998;129:517–524.
10. Glynn, S.A., Albanes, D., Pietinen, P., Brown, C.C., Rautalahti, M., Tangrea, J.A., Gunter, E.W., Barrett, M.J., Virtamo, J., and Taylor, P.R. Colorectal cancer and folate status: a nested case-control study among male smokers. Cancer Epidemiol, Biomarkers Prev 1996;5:487–94.
11. Green, M.S., and Jucha, E. Association of serum lipid with coffee, tea, and egg consumption in free-living subjects. J Epidemiol Comm Health 1986;40:324–29.
12. Hu, F.B., Stampfer, M.J., Rimm, E.B., Manson, J.E. A. Ascherio, G.A. Colditz, B.A. Rosner, D. Spiegelman, F.E. Speizer, F.W. Sacks, C.H. Hennekens, and W.C. Willett. A prospective study of egg consumption and risk of cardiovascular disease in men and women. J Am Med Assoc 1999;281:1387–94.
13. Kantor, L.S. A Dietary Assessment of the U.S. Food Supply. Agricultural Economic Report No. 772. U.S. Department of Agriculture, Economic Research Service, 1998.
14. Kritchevsky, S.B., Tell, G.S., Shimakawa, T., Dennis, B., Li, R., Kohlmeier, L., Steere, E., and Heiss, G. Provitamin carotenoid intake and carotid artery plaques: the atherosclerosis risk in communities study. Am J Clin Nutr 1998;68:726–733.
15. Kushi, L.H., Lew, R.A., Stare, F.J., Ellison, C.R., el Lozy, M., Bourke, G., Daly, L., Graham, I., Hickey, N., and Mulcahy, R. Diet and 20-year mortality from coronary heart disease. N Engl J Med 1985;312:811–18.
16. Landgren, F., Israelsson, B., Lindgren, A., Hultberg, B., Andersson, A., and Brattström, L. Plasma homocysteine in acute myocardial infarction: homocysteine-lowering effect of folic acid. J Intern Med 1995;237:381–88.
17. Life Sciences Research Office (LSRO). Prepared for the Interagency Board for Nutrition Monitoring and Related Research. Third Report on Nutrition Monitoring in the United States: Volume 1. Washington, DC: U.S. Government Printing Office, 1995, 365 pp.

18. Life Sciences Research Office (LSRO). Prepared for the Interagency Board for Nutrition Monitoring and Related Research. Third Report on Nutrition Monitoring in the United States: Volume 2. Washington, DC: U.S. Government Printing Office, 1995, 353 pp.
19. McNamara, DJ. Eggs, dietary cholesterol and heart disease risk: an analysis of experimental and epidemiological data. Report for Egg Nutrition Center, Washington, DC, 1999.
20. MRC Vitamin Study Research Group. Prevention of neural tube defects: results of the Medical Research Council Vitamin Study. Lancet 1991;338:131–37.
21. Riggs, K.M., Apiro, A., III, Tucker, K., and Rush, D. Relations of vitamin B-12, vitamin B-6, folate and homocysteine to cognitive performance in the Normative Aging Study. Am J Clin Nutr 1996;63:306–14.
22. Rimm, E.B, Stampfer, M.J., Ascherio, A., Giovannucci, E., Colditz, G.A., and Willett, W.C. Vitamin E consumption and the risk of coronary heart disease in men. N Engl J Med 1993;328:1450–56.
23. Rimm, E.B., Willett, W.C., Hu, F.B., Sampson, L., Colditz, G.A., Manson, J.E., Hennekens, C., and Stampfer, M.J. Folate and vitamin B_6 from diet and supplements in relation to risk of coronary heart disease among women. J Am Med Assoc 1998;279:359–64.
24. Robinson, K., Arheart, K., Refsum, H., Brattström, L., Boers, G., Ueland, P., Rubba, P., Palma-Reis, R., Meleasy, R., Daly, L., Witteman, J., and Graham, I. Low circulating folate and vitamin B_6 concentrations; risk factors for stroke, peripheral vascular disease, and coronary artery disease. Circulation 1998;97:437–43.
25. Schorah, C.J., Devitt, H., Lucock, M., and Dowell, A.C. The responsiveness of plasma homocysteine to small increases in dietary folic acid; a primary care study. Eur J Clin Nutr 1998;52:407–11.
26. Selhub, J., Jacques, P.F., Wilson, P.W., Rush, D., and Rosenberg, I.H. Vitamin status and intake as primary determinants of homocysteinemia in an elderly population. J Am Med Assoc 1993;270:2693–98.
27. Shaw, G.M., Schaffer, D., Velie, E.M., Morland, K., and Harris, J.A. Periconceptional vitamin use dietary folate, and the occurrence of neural tube defects. Epidemiology 1995;6:219–26.
28. Smithells, R.W., Sheppard, S., and Schorah, C.J. Vitamin deficiencies and neural tube defects. Arch Dis Child 1976;51:944–50.
29. Sommerburg, O., Keunen, J.E., Bird, A.C., and Van Kujik, F.J. Fruits and vegetables that are sources for lutein and zeaxanthin: the macular pigment in human eyes. Br J Ophthamol 1998;82:907–10.
30. Song, W., and Kerver, J. Nutritional contribution of eggs to American diets. J Am Coll Nutr 2000;19:556S–62S.
31. Subar, A.F., Krebs-Smith, S.M., Cook, A., and Kahle, L.L. Dietary sources of nutrients among US adults, 1989 to 1991. J Am Diet Assoc 1998a;98:537–47.
32. Subar, A.F., Krebs-Smith, S.M., Cook, A., and Kahle, L.L. Dietary sources of nutrients among US children, 1989 to 1991. Pediatrics 1998b;102:913–23.
33. Verhoff, P., Stampfer, M.J., Buring, J.E., Gaziano, J.M., Allen, R.H., Stabler, S.P., Reynolds, R.S., Kok, F.J., Hennekens, C.H., and Willett, W.C. Homocysteine metabolism and risk of myocardial infarction: relation with vitamins B_6, B_{12}, and folate. Am J Epidemiol 1996;143:845–59.
34. Vorster, H.H., Bernade, A.J., Barnard, H.C., Locke, M.L., Silvis, N., Venter, C.S., Smuts,

S.M., Endelbrecht, G.P., and Marais, M.P. Egg intake does not change plasma lipoprotein and coagulation profiles. Am J Clin Nutr 1992;55:400–10.

35. Werler, M.M., Shapiro, S., and Mitchell, A.A. Periconceptional folic acid and risk of occurrent neural tube defects. J Am Med Assoc 1993;269:1257–61.

36. Woodside, J.V., Yarnell, J.W., McMaster, D., Young, I.S., Harmon, D.L., McCrum, E.E., Patterson, C.C., Gey, K.F., Whitehead, A.S., and Evans, A. Effect of B-group vitamins and antioxidant vitamins on hyperhomocysteinemia: a double-blind, randomized, factorial-design, controlled trial. Am J Clin Nutr 1998;67:858–66.

3

Designer Eggs: Nutritional and Functional Significance

Jeong S. Sim
and Hoon H. Sunwoo

Consumers' awareness of the relationship between dietary lipid and the incidence of coronary heart disease has changed their attitude toward eggs. Eggs have been singled out as a food to avoid, which has resulted in a significant reduction in egg consumption in many parts of the world. Due to their unsuccessful attempts to significantly reduce egg cholesterol content through genetic, nutritional, and pharmacological tools, researchers have turned toward using the egg as a vehicle for delivering essential nutrients that traditionally were absent or in low concentration in the egg.

The health-promoting effects of dietary omega-3 fatty acids have provoked considerable effort to enrich animal products using various sources of omega-3 fatty acids. The egg industry in particular has been seeking new technology to exploit products beyond their traditional food value. One such technology is Dr. Sim's Canadian Designer Eggs™ (hereafter, referred to as Designer Eggs), which retain their functional, nutritional, and sensory qualities but have a significantly altered lipid composition.

An increased level of long-chain polyunsaturated fatty acids (PUFAs) in foods, however, poses potential risks. Auto-oxidation of PUFAs may occur in animal products. Cholesterol also undergoes auto-oxidation in the presence of light and molecular oxygen through a free-radical reaction. Caution, therefore, is warranted in scaling up the production of omega-3 PUFA–enriched animal products since the susceptibility of animal products to peroxidation is closely associated with the degree of "unsaturation." Little information is available about the stability of egg cholesterol in omega-3 PUFA–enriched eggs. This chapter introduces the Designer Eggs concept and its nutritional and health implications and presents data pertaining to egg lipids and cholesterol stability in omega-3 PUFA–enriched egg yolks and the ways of preventing auto-oxidation.

Introduction

For humans in the industrialized world, animal products contribute more than 60 percent of the total lipids, 70 percent of the saturated fats, and 100 percent of the cholesterol of their diet. Consumer preference for animal products will likely continue. Thus, it would be of strategic importance in the fight against heart disease to design/modify animal products in such a way that dietary risks are minimized. Both epidemiological and clinical intervention studies have demonstrated a decrease of coronary heart disease mortality in people consuming relatively small amounts of omega-3 fatty acids (0.5 g/day) over a long period of time. One large Designer Egg supplies more than 600 mg of most needed omega-3 PUFAs and 6 mg of tocopherols; it would still have additional beneficial effects for egg consumers due to its balanced ratios of PUFAs/SFAs (saturated fatty acids) (1:1) and omega-6/omega-3 PUFAs (1:1). Therefore, Designer Eggs may offer an alternative choice to nutrition and health conscious egg consumers.

Similar efforts should be made to design other animal products that help to minimize the dietary risk of coronary heart disease. Consumers have begun to take control of their own health. They are driving the market for a new category of food with potential health benefits well beyond those traditionally recognized. An increasingly competitive world market environment requires that industry concentrate on producing what the market needs rather than simply supplying what it produces. Designer Egg production has enormous market potential.

Food Lipids and Egg Industry

The rapid decline in per capita consumption of eggs over the past 50 years (Fig. 3.1) is a challenging problem facing the egg industry in many parts of the world. The negative perception related to the high cholesterol content, 195–250 mg/egg,[1] is undoubtedly one of the major contributing factors. Consumers' attitude toward lipid in general has changed their attitude toward egg consumption because of their fear that egg cholesterol will raise their blood cholesterol levels. Therefore, eggs have been singled out as a food to avoid[2] even though the egg contains the best and least expensive high-quality protein and balanced distribution of minerals and vitamins, except vitamin C.[3]

The first response to "cholesterol phobia" was the extensive investigation into factors, genetic, dietary, and pharmacological in nature, that would reduce the cholesterol content of eggs.[4] However, various attempts to reduce the cholesterol content[5] or produce cholesterol-free products have met with no success. Due to the lack of success in attempts to significantly reduce cholesterol levels in the egg, researchers began to investigate alternative manipulation to improve the nutritional quality of the egg and re-establish its position as a healthy and safe food item.

Advocates for reducing egg consumption point out that the amount and type of dietary lipids influence plasma and lipoprotein lipid levels, which in turn, increase the risk of coronary heart disease.[6] The principal nutrient-related health problems in North America

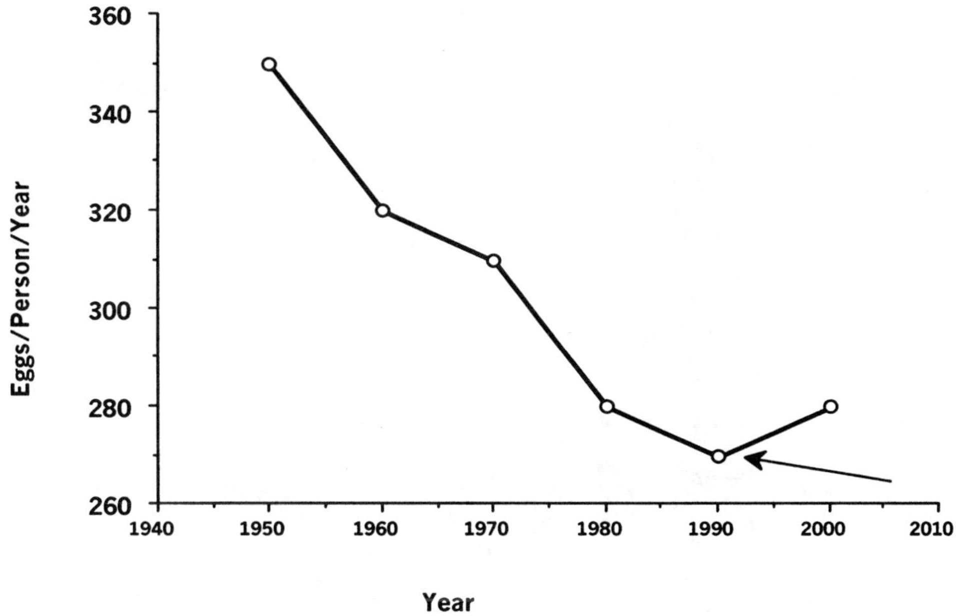

Figure 3.1. Egg consumption pattern in the United States during the last 50 years. Now, the declining trend of egg consumption has been reversed in North America and has begun to rise since 1996 (*arrow*). This change has been attributed to the new market surge of specialty eggs, like Designer Eggs.

arise from the overconsumption of lipid, mainly of animal origin (57–75 percent). The National Institutes of Health[7] and Health Canada[8] have adopted recommendations and target dietary guidelines to limit lipid intake and modify the type of lipid consumption (Fig. 3.2). Thus, animal agriculture must respond to the perceived needs of consumers by producing foods that follow national nutritional guidelines. The egg industry in particular has been greatly encouraged to intensify efforts in developing and marketing products that would facilitate consumers' adherence to the dietary guidelines or national recommended target levels for fat and cholesterol.

Omega-3 Fatty Acids

The pioneering discovery that omega-3 fatty acids protect against coronary heart disease in Greenland Eskimos consuming fish[9] has generated much research on the various health benefits of dietary omega-3 fatty acids from fish oils. Researchers around the world have focused on the health effects of the dietary supply of omega-3 fatty acids, partly because those fatty acids have been reported to protect against cardiovascular and inflammatory diseases, as well as certain types of cancer[10,11] and partly because it has been shown that omega-3 fatty acids are essential nutrients for adults and children.[12,13] The benefits of dietary omega-3 PUFAs include, among others, reduction in plasma triglycerides, blood pressure, platelet aggregation, thrombosis and atherosclerosis particularly in diabetics, tumor growth, and skin disease and enhanced immunity. The Canadian government[8]

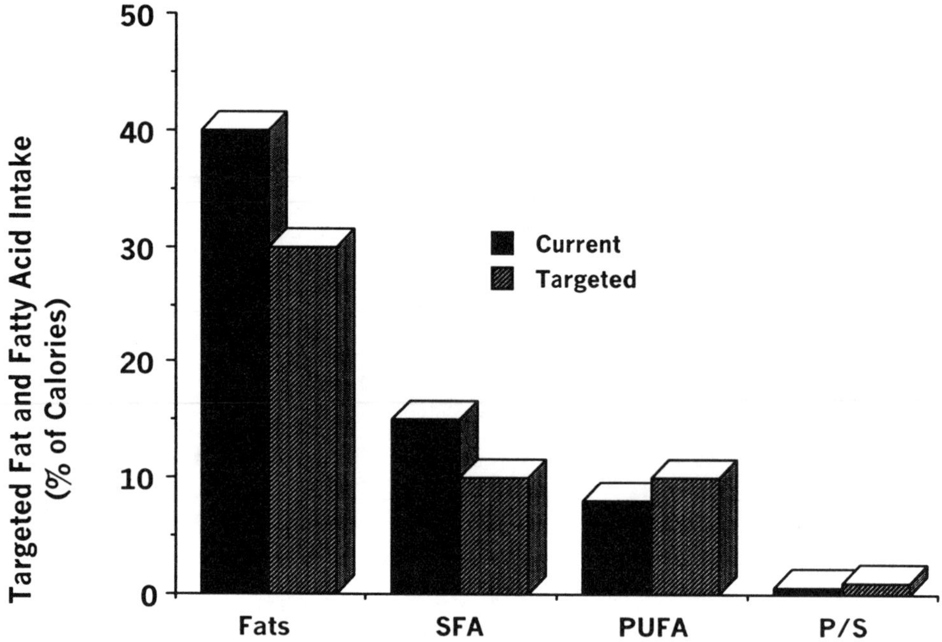

Figure 3.2. National Health Organization recommended dietary guidelines. It suggests reducing total fat intake to less than 30 percent of total calories, SFA intake to less than 10 percent, and PUFA intake to 10 percent of total caloric intake. SFA = saturated fatty acids, PUFA = polyunsaturated fatty acid, and P/S = polyunsaturated/saturated.

adopted a recommendation that omega-3 PUFAs are essential, thus recommending that the dietary supply should be at least 0.5 percent of the energy intake as α-linolenic acid (α-LNA). When the diet of infants contains no eicosapentanoic acid (EPA) and docosahexanoic acid (DHA), then α-LNA should be supplied as 1 percent of energy intake. This recommendation was based on the fact that North American diets are depleted of the omega-3 fatty acids.

The egg industry has stepped in to fill this gap and has begun to return the omega-3 fatty acids into the food supply. The ratio of omega-6 to omega-3 fatty acids is important, and the current high ratio in human diets should be reduced to less than 4 to 1.[14] To date, the main supply of omega-3 fatty acids in the human diet has been fish and fish oil. The major omega-6 and omega-3 PUFAs are summarized in Table 3.1.

Designer Eggs

The fatty acid composition of yolk fat can readily be modified by changing the chicken's diet.[15,16] In recent years several researchers have investigated the ability of the hen to enrich the egg with omega-3 fatty acids. The incorporation of omega-3 PUFAs into egg yolk fat was easily accomplished by feeding laying hens diets containing flaxseed[17–20] and

Table 3.1. Major omega-6 and omega-3 fatty acids

Omega-6 Fatty acids	
Linoleic acid (LA)	C18:2ω6
Arachidonic acid (AA)	C20:4ω6
Omega-3 Fatty acids	
Linolenic acid (LNA)	C18:3ω3
Eicosapentanoic acid (EPA)	C20:5ω3
Docosapentanoic acid (DPA)	C22:5ω3
Docosahexanoic acid (DHA)	C22:6ω3

fish oils.[21,22] The egg lipid composition is the result of a combination of de novo lipogenesis and incorporation of lipid components from the diet. Another factor regulating the quantity and the type of fatty acid deposition is the feedback inhibition of dietary long-chain PUFAs.[23] Therefore, it is feasible to alter the fatty acid composition of poultry products through dietary manipulation of long-chain PUFAs and to design food products meeting the nutritional guidelines, supplying omega-3 fatty acids while having optimal PUFAs:SFAs and omega-6:omega-3 fatty acid ratios.

Our research group[24–26] has carried out a series of studies to enhance the value of chicken eggs by enriching them in omega-3 fatty acids (500–600 mg/egg) with a significantly elevated PUFAs:SFAs ratio (from 0.6 to 1.02) and lowering the omega-6:omega-3 fatty acid ratio (from 10:1 to 1:1) (Fig. 3.3). One large egg can supply about 600 mg of total omega-3 fatty acids (balanced with DHA, docosapentanoic acid [DPA], and EPA) equivalent to an approximately 100 g serving of fish. A consumer survey indicated the public's interest in omega-3 fatty acid enriched eggs as a dietary alternative to fish.[27]

Although α-LNA was the major omega-3 fatty acid deposited in the egg yolk, a considerable amount of longer-chain omega-3 fatty acids were also incorporated into the phospholipid fractions of the yolk lipids. The hens fed flaxseed produced eggs enriched with omega-3 fatty acids (7–12 percent of yolk lipids) in the following order: α-LNA > DHA > DPA >EPA.[28] This indicates that laying hens can convert dietary α-LNA to EPA, DPA and DHA via the desaturase and elongase enzyme systems.[29] Arachidonic acid (AA), the metabolite of linoleic acid (omega-6 fatty acid), was significantly reduced. Consequently, the ratio of omega-6 to omega-3 fatty acid was significantly decreased in the omega-3 fatty acid–enriched eggs (from 10:1 to 1:1).

Nutritional Significance

A series of studies was carried out to examine the influence, if any, omega-3 PUFA–enriched eggs have on plasma cholesterol and tissue fatty acid modification in animals and humans. Plasma and liver tissue cholesterol levels and fatty acid composition were analyzed after feeding omega-3 fatty acid–enriched eggs to rats,[30] as animal models, and humans,[31] as egg consumers.

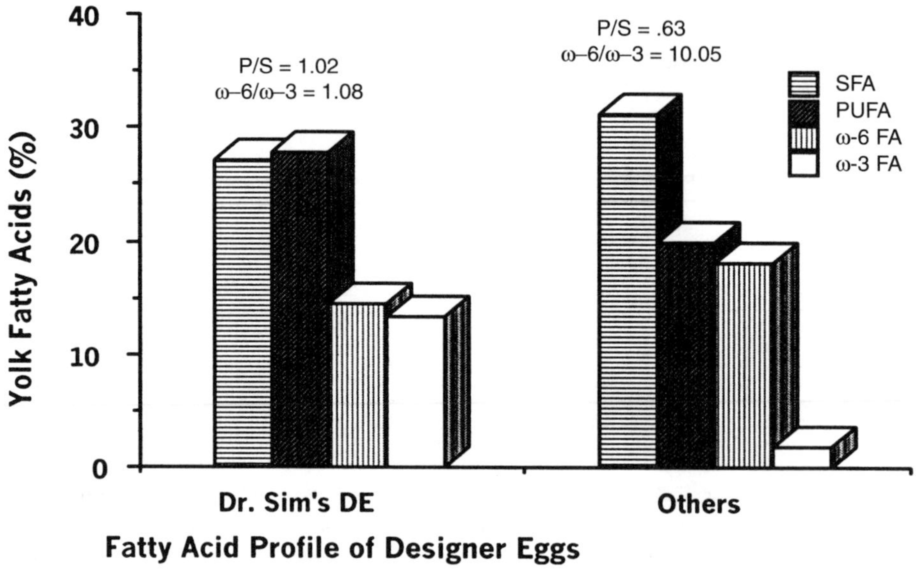

Figure 3.3. Fatty acid profile comparison of Designer Eggs (DE) and regular egg (others). P/S = polyunsaturated/saturated, SFA = saturated fatty acid, PUFA = polyunsaturated fatty acid, ω-6 FA = omega-6 fatty acids, and ω-3 FA = omega-3 fatty acid.

Plasma Lipids

The eggs were hard-boiled, and yolks were removed, pulverized, and dried. Dry yolk powders were incorporated into a semisynthetic diet at a 15 percent level and fed to weaning female Sprague-Dawley rats for 4 weeks. The blood and liver cholesterol levels and fatty acid composition were determined at the end of the feeding period. Feeding omega-3 PUFA–enriched eggs reduced both plasma and liver total cholesterol contents by 20 and 38 percent, respectively (Fig. 3.4).

Twenty-four healthy male students aged 18–32 were recruited and randomly divided into two groups of 12 each. Each subject had two eggs at breakfast. Before the start and at the termination of the 18-day study, subjects fasted for more than 12 hours to take blood samples at the university health clinic. There are clear patterns that indicate that consumption of Designer Eggs (1) does not increase plasma cholesterol despite their high inherent cholesterol content, (2) increases HDL (high-density lipoprotein) cholesterol, (3) suppresses LDL (low-density lipoprotein) cholesterol, and (4) produces a marked reduction of plasma triglyceride levels (Fig. 3.5). Consuming Designer Eggs also enriches body tissue lipids with omega-3 fatty acids, in particular phospholipids. Similar results were reported by Ferrier et al.,[32] who found that human consumption of α-LNA–enriched eggs decreased serum triglycerides and increased omega-3 fatty acids, particularly DHA, which accumulated in platelet phospholipids.

The results demonstrate that the cholesterolemic and lipidemic properties of chicken eggs can be modified by "designing" the fatty acid composition of egg yolk lipids through chicken diets. Designer Eggs offer an alternative to nutrition conscious consumers around

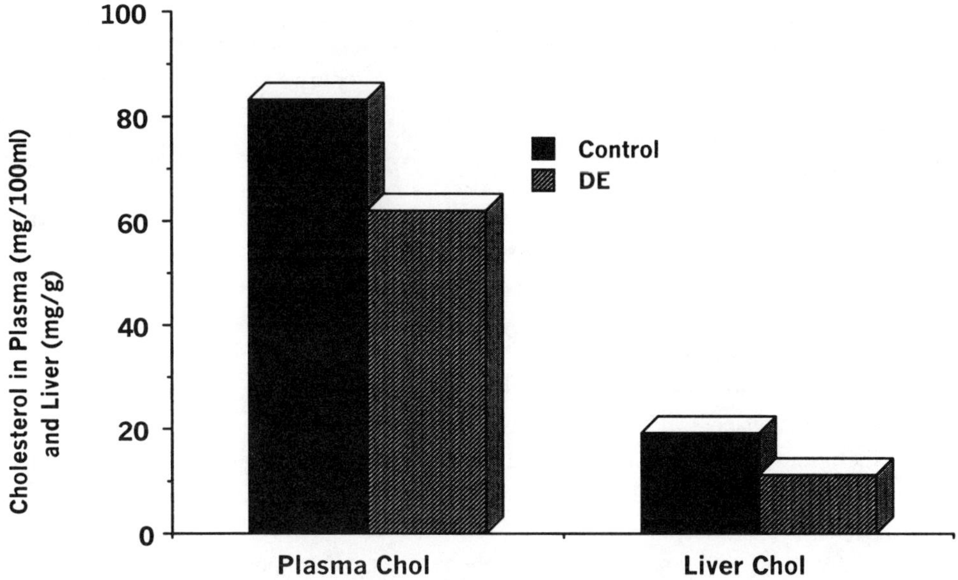

Figure 3.4. Plasma and liver cholesterol levels of rats at the end of 28 days of being fed yolk powder with and without omega-3 PUFA enrichment. DE = Designer Eggs.

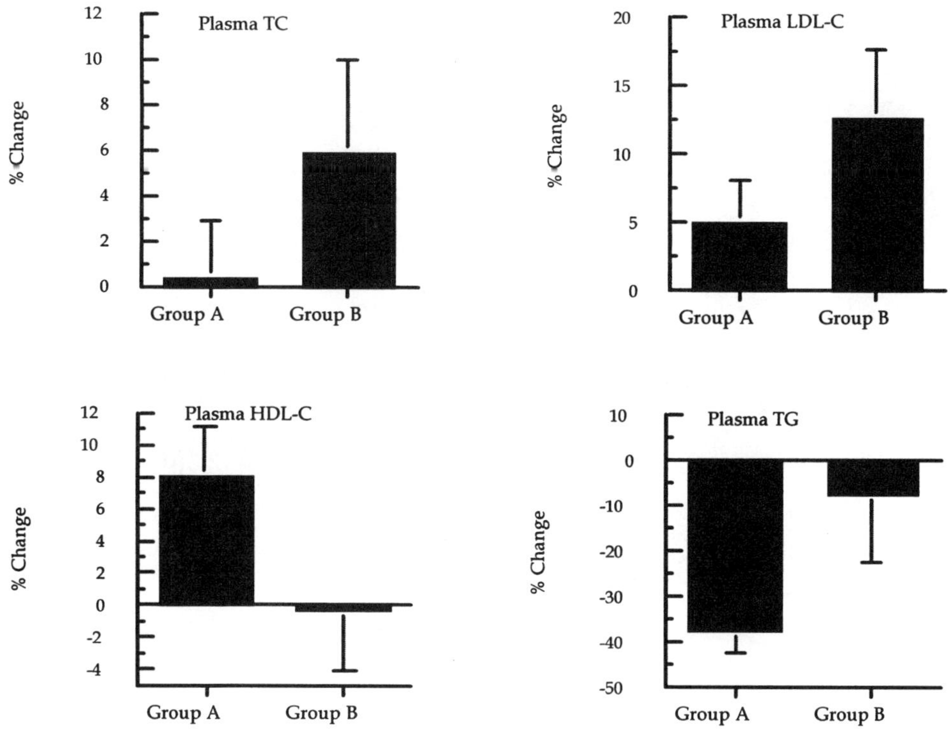

Figure 3.5. Percentage change in plasma total cholesterol (TC), low-density lipoprotein cholesterol (LDL-C), high-density lipoprotein cholesterol (HDL-C), and plasma triglyceride (TG) levels in human subjects after consuming two Designer Eggs (A) or regular eggs (B) with their habitual diets for a period of 3 weeks.

the world. Eggs have long been considered an atherogenic food but are not if enriched with omega-3 fatty acids.

Mother's Milk

Aware of the importance of omega-3 PUFAs to infants, Carlson et al. studied the magnitude of changes in the fatty acid composition of breast milk and plasma fatty acids of eight nursing women upon consumption of two Designer Eggs for a period of 6 weeks.[33] Consuming two Designer Eggs as a part of their normal daily meal for 6 weeks resulted in a significant deposition of total omega-3 fatty acids at 3.6 percent compared with 1.9 percent for the pretest milk and a reduction in the omega-6:omega-3 fatty acid ratio from 6.7 to 3. The longer-chain EPA and DHA comprised 1.2 percent compared with 0.4 percent in the pretest milk. Consuming omega-3–enriched eggs did not alter the AA content in the milk. This phenomenon made the milk fat more favorable by increasing the DHA to AA ratio from 0.75 to 1.2 (Fig. 3.6). Total plasma cholesterol and triglyceride levels were not affected.[34] The omega-3 PUFA–enriched eggs (Designer Eggs) contained about 690 mg of total omega-3 fatty acid with 165 mg of long-chain n-3 fatty acids (EPA, DPA, and DHA). If the intake of a 1-month-old infant is assumed to be 794 ml, infants nursed from women consuming Designer Eggs could have over 300 mg of long-chain omega-3

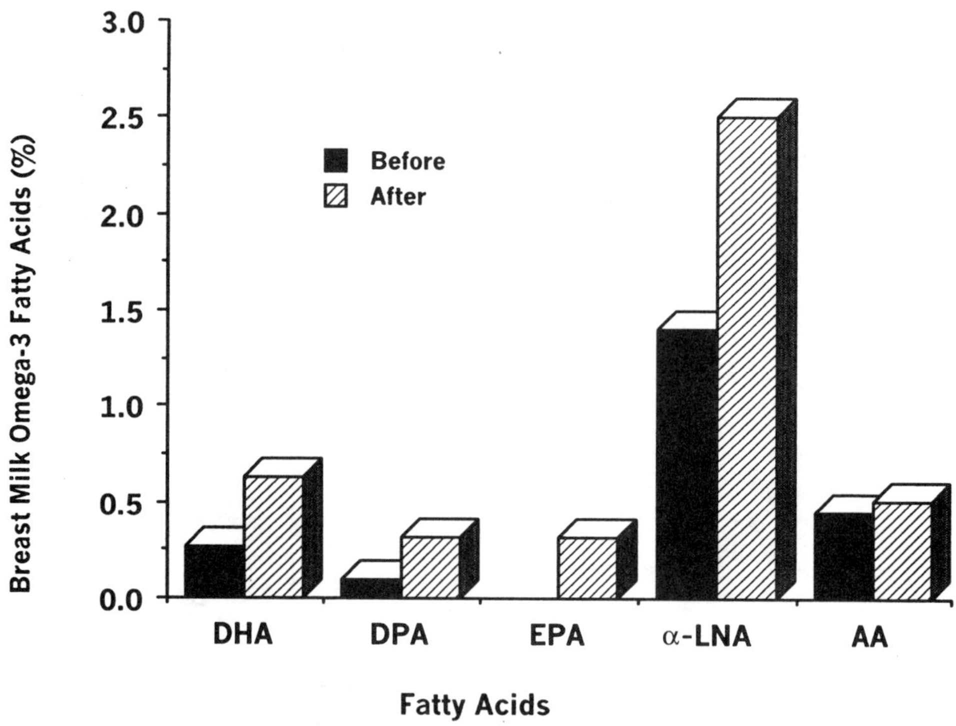

Figure 3.6. Fatty acid composition of breast milk from nursing mothers before (basal) and after (6th week) consuming two Designer Eggs daily for a period of 6 weeks. DHA = docosahexanoic acid, DPA = docosapentanoic acid, EPA = eicosapentanoic acid, α-LNA = α-linolenic acid, and AA = arachidonic acid.

fatty acids such as EPA, DPA, and DHA. Thus, a diet supplemented with Designer Eggs or their egg oils should provide an alternative way of supplying omega-3 fatty acids to breast-fed infants. These differences in the omega-3 fatty acid content of breast milk could have implications for the development of suckling infants.

Infant Food Oils

The egg yolk consists of lipids and protein. More than 66 percent of the total dry yolk mass is fats. An average egg provides about 6 g of lipids, which are contained exclusively in the yolk. With elevated levels of DHA and AA, one Designer Egg can supply about 600 mg of total omega-3 PUFAs to the human diet. Both the DHA and AA are essential for proper brain development of infants.[35] The Designer Egg is a potential vehicle to provide the much needed DHA and AA, which more closely mimics the fatty acid composition of human breast milk (Fig. 3.7). In contrast to human milk, most commercial infant formulas are based on soybean oil and contain about 53 percent linoleic acid (LA) and 7 percent α-LNA. Most infant formulas contain LA and α-LNA in amounts comparable to those in human milk, but they lack long-chain omega-3 PUFA contents, DHA and AA in particular.[36] It is crucially important to supply the preformed essential long-chain PUFAs, both omega-3 DHA and omega-6 AA, in an adequate balance.[33] Currently available infant formulas do not contain fatty acids above 18 carbons (Table 3.2). The primary goal of infant formulas is that the formula-fed infant grows and develops like the breast-fed.[36] One approach to improve a milk formula is to match the composition of human breast milk, which contains both DHA and AA (Fig. 3.7). Designer Egg yolk oils provide an adequate amount of omega-3 and omega-6 precursors and long-chain PUFAs, including DHA, while still sustaining a significant level of AA in the egg with various ratios of omega-6/omega-3 ranging from 20 to 1. Industry and the scientific community alike are searching for a new oil source supplying both long-chain omega-6 and omega-3 PUFAs. Since the fatty acid makeup of Designer Eggs resembles that of human milk fat, yolk oil may be regarded as an essential oil base for infant food industry.

Table 3.2. Essential fatty acid profile of commercial infant formulas, Designer Egg oils, and human breast milk (survey conducted)

	Commercial infant formulas (%)					DE oils (%)	HBM (%)
LA	13.9	22.0	23.6	31.2	31.1	13.0	9.9
LNA	1.9	3.1	3.5	4.4	4.1	9.3	2.4
AA	—	—	—	—	—	1.6	0.4
DHA	—	—	—	—	—	2.2	0.3

Note. LA = linoleic acid (18:2ω6), LNA = linolenic acid (18:3ω3), AA = arachidonic acid (20:4ω6), DHA = docosahexanoic acid (22:6ω3), DE = Designer Egg, HBM = human breast milk.

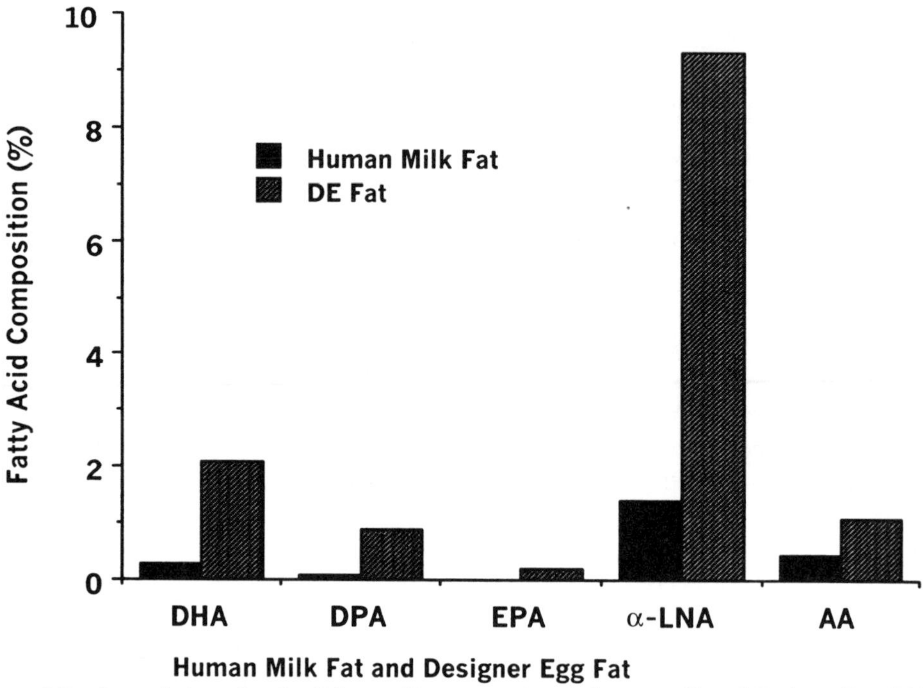

Figure 3.7. Long-chain ω-6 and ω-3 fatty acid concentrations in human milk and Designer Egg (DE) oil. DHA = docosahexanoic acid, DPA = docosapentanoic acid, EPA = eicosapentanoic acid, α-LNA = α-linolenic acid, and AA = arachidonic acid.

Designer Egg Oil

An average egg also provides about 6 g of lipids, which are contained exclusively in the yolk. More than 66 percent of the total yolk mass is fats; thus, the yolk from these n-3 PUFA–enriched eggs can be regarded as a potential oil crop rich in long-chain PUFAs, both the DHA and AA essential for infants. Designer egg yolk oil may be regarded as an essential oil base for infant formula because it resembles the fatty acid composition of human milk. Designed egg yolk oils provide an adequate amount of n-3 and n-6 precursors and long-chain PUFAs including DHA still sustaining a significant level of AA in the egg with various ratios of n-6/n-3 in a range of 22.1 to 1.4.

Egg oil extraction-purification technologies developed at the University of Alberta are available that can be adopted by industry. A bench top model of technology for extracting oil directly from fresh egg yolk using an aqueous solvent system and subsequently partitioning into the neutral oil and lecithin fractions by a cold precipitation technique was devised and patented as a potential technology to be exploited by industry (Fig. 3.8). Later, a scaled-up process was jointly undertaken in collaboration with food industry partners (technology of egg oil extraction and fractionation of lecithin) from fresh egg yolk (Canadian Patent Application No. 612,411, September 21, 1989, European Patents, Japan, South Korea, Finland under patent cooperation treaty, PCT No. 8150, July 10, 1990).

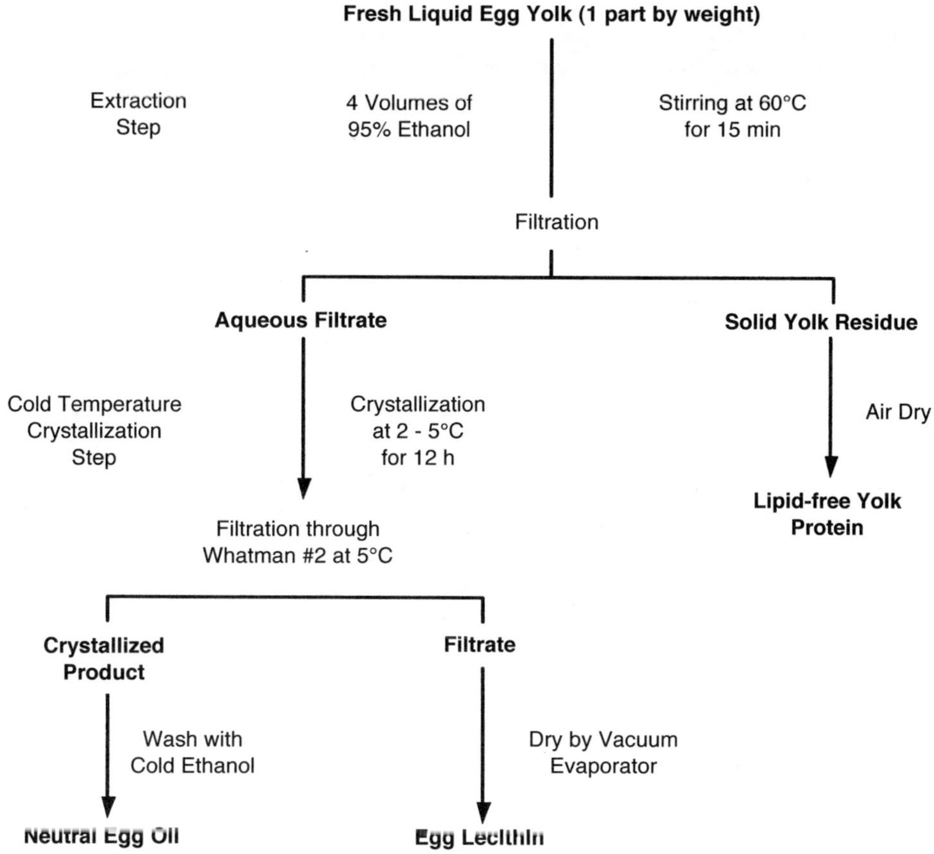

Figure 3.8. Schematic flow chart of sequential extraction, fractionation, and purification procedure for egg oil and lecithin from fresh yolk.

Oxidative Stability

There are potential risks associated with a high level of long-chain PUFAs in foods. Auto-oxidation of long-chain PUFAs occurs in feeds and egg products. Caution is warranted in scaling up the production of omega-3 PUFA–enriched eggs, egg oils, and their infant food applications, since the susceptibility of food lipids to oxidation is closely associated with the degree of unsaturation. A series of experiments to investigate the lipid stability from lipid oxidation and ways of preventing auto-oxidation has been conducted.

Chicken Feed

In an earlier study, feeds containing large amounts of flaxseed were associated with a fish flavor or lower sensory quality of egg products during storage. This was attributed to a combination of lipid rancidity in the feed and lipid peroxidation in the chicken tissues and eggs.[37] Therefore, Gopalakrishnan et al. conducted an experiment to monitor the chemical changes in the flaxseed, the very source of dietary omega-3 fatty acid in the poultry feed under various storage conditions. The changes in the content and stability of α-LNA were found negligible in the early stage of storage, but oxidation potential markedly increased after 60 days. Results indicated that the intact (whole) flaxseed is well protected from lipid oxidation by the presence of its intrinsic tocopherol content, and further supplementation of tocopherol significantly extends its stability even when the flaxseed is physically broken open for feed compounding and storage. This study confirmed that flaxseed contains a sufficient amount of natural antioxidants as tocopherols that protect dietary omega-3 fatty acids in the chicken feed from auto-oxidation within 60 days.[38]

Antioxidants: Tocopherols

In an early stage of development, Designer Eggs enriched with omega-3 PUFAs had an off-flavor (fish taint). We suspected that the fish flavor could have been the result of rancidity of omega-3 fatty acids either in feeds and/or animal products. This problem was dealt with by stabilizing the dietary source of omega-3 PUFAs with a natural form of tocopherols before incorporating into chicken feeds.[39] A significant reduction in off-flavor, volatile compounds, cholesterol oxidation products, and thiobarbituric acid (TBA) –reacting substances was achieved in both feed and egg products by stabilizing the dietary fats before incorporating them into chicken feed with a natural form of tocopherols as antioxidants.[40–42] Supplementing antioxidants into chicken feed not only effectively eliminates the off-flavor problem but also greatly improves the stability of egg products. The toco-

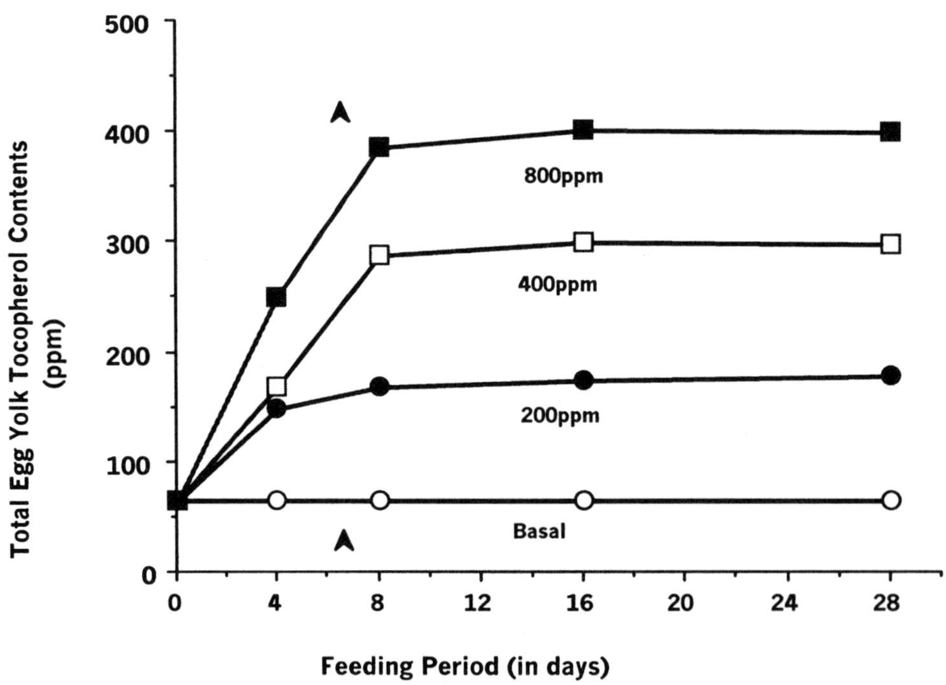

Figure 3.9. Supplementation of natural tocopherols at various levels into chicken feed reaches a plateau on the 8th day of feeding. Tocopherol deposition into the egg yolk is proportional to the dietary levels.

pherol concentrations of egg yolk increased linearly with increasing levels of dietary tocopherol levels (Fig. 3.9).

With increasing levels of dietary tocopherol supplementation in laying hen diets, malondialdehyde contents in the egg yolk decreased from 41 to 18 nmol/g of egg yolk (Fig. 3.10). This proves that lipid stability could be improved by increasing the tocopherol content of eggs. Reduction of the oxidation products and increasing the tocopherol concentration (antioxidants) in the yolk were major technological breakthroughs that eliminated sensory and off-flavor problems. Thus, Designer Eggs not only supply a stable form of essential omega-3 PUFAs but also a natural form of tocopherols, including Vitamin E, to health conscious consumers.

Cholesterol Oxidation

Through a free-radical reaction, cholesterol undergoes auto-oxidation in the presence of light and molecular oxygen and forms cholesterol oxide products that are considered potent atherogens and carcinogens to humans.[43,44] The presence of several cholesterol oxide products in commercial egg products has been reported, but little information about cholesterol stability in omega-3 fatty acid–enriched eggs and means of prevention is available. Considering the importance of PUFAs and tocopherols as antioxidants in lipid oxidation, researchers investigated feeding laying hens flax, sunflower, palm, and fish oils (with and without tocopherols) and their effect on the oxidative stability of cholesterol in the egg yolk. Results show that cholesterol oxidation is accelerated by the presence of long-chain PUFAs in the order of fish oil > flaxseed oil > sunflower seed oil > palm oil.

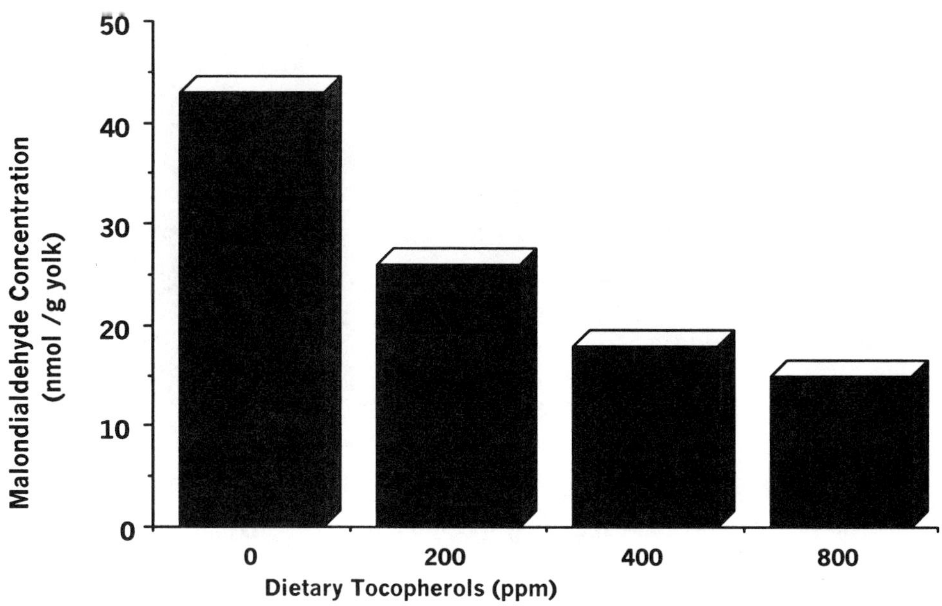

Figure 3.10. Effect of tocopherol supplementation on lipoperoxide level in the egg yolk. Egg yolk lipid stability was greatly improved by increasing tocopherol contents of eggs.

The initial levels of cholesterol oxides were 7-10 ppm and reached over 200 ppm within a 4-month storage period. Cholesterol oxide formation was further accelerated by heat at 110°C for 22 hours. Feeding tocopherol supplements to laying hens increased intrinsic tocopherol content in eggs, and the presence of increased tocopherols significantly reduced the formation of cholesterol oxides in the egg yolk regardless of its fatty acid profiles (Fig 3.11). Feeding laying hens tocopherol-supplemented diets can delay or prevent the cholesterol oxidation of Designer Eggs during storage and processing. This study suggests that cholesterol oxide formation in Designer Eggs can be prevented by adding Vitamin E or a natural form of tocopherols, which would benefit the food industry and human health.

Acknowledgments

Research for this chapter was supported by grants from the Natural Sciences Engineering Research Council of Canada (NSERC), University of Alberta, Alberta Agricultural Research Institute (AARI), Flax Council of Canada, and Designer Egg Producers Association International (DEPAI).

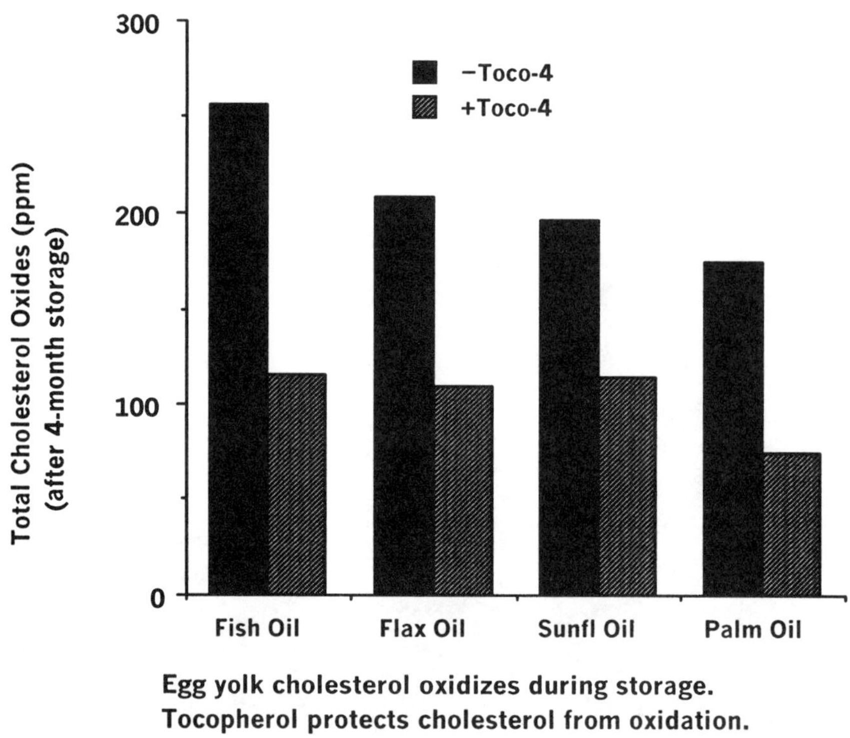

Figure 3.11. Effects of dietary fatty acids and tocopherol supplementation on cholesterol oxidation in the egg yolk. The cholesterol oxidation was significantly reduced in the presence of tocopherol.

References

1. Yaffee, M., Schultz, H., Stone, J., Brokhari, S., and Zeidler, G. Consumer perception and utilization of eggs and egg products. Poult Sci 1991;70:188–92.
2. Connor, S.L., and Connor, W.E. The importance of dietary cholesterol in coronary heart disease. Prev Med 1983;12:115.
3. Shrimpton, D.H. The nutritive value of eggs and their dietary significance. In Egg Quality—Current Problems and Recent Advances, Wells, R.G., and Beljavin, C.G., eds. London: Butterworth and Co., Ltd., 1987, pp. 11–25.
4. Hargis, P.S. Modifying egg cholesterol in the domestic fowl: A review. World's Poult Sci 1988;44:17–29.
5. Waldroup P.W., Ndife, L.I., Hellwig, H.M., Herbert, J.A., and Berrio, L. Influence of probuccal on egg cholesterol concentration. Poult Sci 1986;64:205–11.
6. U.S. Department of Health and Human Services. The Surgeon General's report on nutrition and health. Washington, DC: U.S. Government Printing Office, 1988.
7. National Institutes of Health. NIH Consensus Development Statement on Lowering Blood Cholesterol to Prevent Heart Disease. Vol. 5, no. 7. National Institutes of Health, Washington, DC, 1984.
8. Health Canada. Nutritional Recommendations. Ottawa: Canadian Government Publishing Centre, 1990, pp. 24, 57.
9. Dyerberg, J., and Bang, H.O. Haemostic function and platelet polyunsaturated fatty acids in Eskimos. Lancet 1979;ii:433–35.
10. Simopoulos, A.P. Omega-3 fatty acids in health and disease and in growth and development. Am J Clin Nutr 1991;54:438–63.
11. Kinsella, J.E., Lokesh, B., and Stone, R.A. Dietary n-3 polyunsaturated fatty acids and amelioration of cardiovascular disease: Possible mechanisms. Am J Clin Nutr 1990;52:1–28.
12. Bjerve, K.S. Omega-3 fatty acid deficiency in man: Implications for requirement of α-linolenic acid and long chain omega-3 fatty acids. In Health effects of omega-3 PUFA in seafoods, Simopoulos, A.P., Kifer, R.R., and Barlow, S.M., eds. World Rev Nutr Diet 1991;65: 133–42.
13. Holman, R.T., Johnson, S.B., and Hatch, T. A case of human linolenic acid deficiency involving neurological abnormalities. Am J Clin Nutr 1982;35:617–23.
14. Beare-Rogers, J. Nutrition recommendations in Canada, Bureau of Nutritional Sciences. Food Directorate, Health Protection Branch, Health and Welfare Canada. Inform 1991;2(4):326. AOCS Annual Meeting at Chicago.
15. Cruickshank, E.M. Studies in fat metabolism in the fowl. In The composition of the egg fat and depot fat of the fowl as affected by the ingestion of large amounts of fats. Biochem J 1934;28:965–71.
16. Sim, J.S., Hudgson, G.S., and Bragg, D.B. Effect of dietary animal tallow and vegetable oil on fatty acid composition of egg yolk, adipose tissue and liver of laying hens. Poult Sci 1973;52:51–57.
17. Nwokolo, E., and Sim, J.S. Barley and full-fat Canola seed in layer diets. Poult Sci 1989;68:1485–89.
18. Sim, J.S. Flaxseed as a high energy/protein/omega-3 fatty acid ingredient for poultry. In Proceedings of the 53rd Flax Institute of the United States, Carter, J.R., ed. Fargo, ND: NDSU, 1990, pp. 65–71.

19. Caston, L., and Leeson, S. Research note: Dietary flaxseed and egg composition. Poult Sci 1990;69:1617–20.
20. Jiang, Z., Ahn, D.U., Ladner, L., and Sim, J.S. Influence of feeding full fat flax and sunflower seeds on internal and sensory qualities of eggs. Poult Sci 1992;71:378–82.
21. Yu, M.M., and Sim, J.S. Biological incorporation of N-polyunsaturated fatty acids into chicken eggs. Poult Sci 1987;66:195 (abstract).
22. Hargis, P.S., van Elswyk, M.E., and Harris, M.M. Dietary modification of yolk lipid with menhaden oil. Poult Sci 1991;70:874–83.
23. Reiser, R., Williams, M.C., Sorrels, M.F., and Murty, N.L. Biosynthesis of fatty acids and cholesterol as related to diet fat. Arch Biochem Biophys 1963;102:276–85.
24. Sim, J.S., Cherian, G., and Jiang, Z. Alpha-linolenic acid metabolism: The chicken and the egg. Int J Appl Basic Nutr Sci (Nutrition) 1992;8:221–22.
25. Jiang, Zhirong, and Sim, Jeong S. Effects of dietary N-3 fatty acid-enriched chicken eggs on plasma and tissue cholesterol and fatty acid compositions of rats. Lipids 1992;27:279–84.
26. Sim, J.S. Designing eggs and health/nutritional implication for egg consumers. Proceedings of 54th Minnesota Nutrition Conference and National Renders Technical Symposium, Bloomington, MN, 1993. pp. 275–86.
27. Marshall, A.C., Kubena, K.S., Hinton, K.R., Hargis, P.S., and van Elswyk, M.E. n-3 Fatty acid enriched table eggs: A survey of consumer acceptability. Poult Sci 1994;73:1334–40.
28. Sim, J.S., and Qi, Guang-Hai. Designing poultry products using flaxseed. In Flaxseed in Human Nutrition, Thompson, L.U., and Cunnane, S., eds. American Oil Chemist's Society Press (AOCS), 1995, pp. 315–33.
29. Garg, M., Sebokova, L.E., Wierzbicki, E., Thompson, A.B.R., and Clandinin, M.T. Differential effects of dietary linoleic and linolenic acid on lipid metabolism in rat tissues. Lipids 1988;23:847–52.
30. Jiang, Zhirong, and S. Sim, Jeong. Effects of dietary n-3 fatty acid-enriched chicken eggs on plasma and tissue cholesterol and fatty acid compositions of rats. Lipids 1992;27:279–84.
31. Jiang, Zhirong, and Sim, Jeong S. Consumption of n-3 fatty acid enriched eggs and changes in plasma lipids of human subjects. Nutrition 1993;9:513–18.
32. Ferrier, L.K., Caston, L., Leeson, S., Squires, E.J., Celi, B., Thomas, L., and Holub, B. Changes in serum lipids and platelet fatty acid composition following consumption of eggs enriched in alpha-linolenic acid (LnA). Food Res Int 1992;25:263–68.
33. Carlson, S.E., Cooke, R.J., Werkman, S.H., and Tolley, E.A. First year growth of infants fed standard compared to marine oil n-3 supplemented formula. Lipids 1992;27:901–7.
34. Cherian, G., and Sim, J.S. Changes in the breast milk fatty acids and plasma lipids of nursing mothers following consumption of n-3 polyunsaturated fatty acid enriched eggs. Nutrition 1996;12:8–12.
35. Cherian, G., Gopalarkrishnan, N., Akiba, Y., and Sim, J.S. Effect of maternal dietary n-3 fatty acids on the accretion of long chain polyunsaturated fatty acids in the tissues of developing chick embryo. Biol Neonate 1997;72:165–74.
36. Simopoulos, A.P., and N. Salem. Egg yolk as a source of long chain polyunsaturated fatty acids in infant feeding. Am J Clin Nutr 1992;55:411–15.
37. Jiang, Zhirong, Ahn, D.U., Ladner, L., and Sim, J.S. Influence of feeding full-fat flax and sunflower seeds on internal and sensory qualities of eggs. Poult Sci 1992;71:378–82.
38. Gopalakrishnan, N., Cherian, G., and Sim, J.S. Chemical changes in the lipids of canola and flax seeds during storage. Fett (Lipid) 1996;98:(Nr.5. S.) 168–71.

39. Qi, G.H., and Sim, J.S. Natural tocopherol enrichment and its effect in n-3 fatty acid modified chicken eggs. J Agric Food Chem 1998;46:1920–26.
40. Li, S.X., Cherian, G., and Sim, J.S. Cholesterol oxidation in egg yolk powder during storage and heating as affected by dietary oils and tocopherol. J Food Sci 1996;61:721–25.
41. Cherian, G., Wolfe, F.W., and Sim, J.S. Dietary oils with added tocopherols: Effects on egg or tissue tocopherols, fatty acids and oxidative stability. Poult Sci 1996;75:423–32.
42. Cherian, G., Wolfe, F.W., and Sim, J.S. Feeding dietary oils with tocopherols: Effects on internal qualities of eggs during storage. J Food Sci 1996;61:15–18.
43. Hubbard, R.W., Ono, Y., and Sanchez, A. Atherogenic effect of oxidized products of cholesterol. Prog Food Nutr Sci 1989;13:17–44.
44. Ames, B.N. Dietary carcinogens and anticarcinogens. Science 1983;221:1256–64.

4

Specialty Eggs: n-3 Fatty Acid–Enriched Eggs

Elizabeth H. Sheppard

INTRODUCTION

Hen eggs contain all the necessary nutrients for the growth of a chicken embryo and are considered a high-quality food for human use. However, in the past 20 years there has been a trend of limiting egg consumption as a way of controlling dietary cholesterol, a known risk of cardiovascular disease. The egg industry has launched several campaigns to reclaim its lost market by introducing low-cholesterol eggs and lower-fat eggs.[2,3,5] The latest and most promising attempt is the introduction of n-3 fatty acid–enriched eggs. These eggs are developed naturally by manipulating the hen's diet to increase the yolk's n-3 fatty acid content.

Concurrently, mounting evidence exists regarding the beneficial effects of increased dietary intake of n-3 fatty acids. n-3 Fatty acids decrease the risk of coronary artery disease and play an important role in the prevention and treatment of hypertension, arthritis, and other autoimmune disorders.[21] n-3 Fatty acids inhibit certain cancers such as breast and prostate[15], delay loss of immunological functions, and are essential for fetal brain and visual development.[12] Of particular importance is the dietary ratio of n-6 fatty acids to n-3 fatty acids. The current Western dietary intake ratio of n-6 to n-3 fatty acids is 20–30:1, which is considerably higher than the suggested ratio of 1–2:1.[20] The low dietary intake of n-3 fatty acid is partially due to reduced fish consumption and to the high n-6 fatty acid content of animal feed, which in turn produces meats and eggs rich in n-6 but low in n-3 fatty acids. n-3 Fatty acid specialty eggs, therefore, may prove to be a healthful and convenient dietary source of n-3 fatty acids for the general population, especially pregnant or lactating women.[4]

ESSENTIAL FATTY ACIDS: FUNCTIONS AND PATHWAYS

Linoleic acid (LA; 18:2n-6) and α-linolenic acid (α-LNA; 18:3n-3) belong, respectively, to the n-6 and n-3 fatty acid families of unsaturated fatty acids. The *n* or ω refers to the position of the first double bond counted from the terminal methyl carbon of the fatty acid.[30] The human body cannot synthesize fatty acids with double bonds between the ninth carbon and the terminal methyl carbon of the fatty acid chain.[30] Therefore, both linoleic acid and α-linolenic acid are essential fatty acids (EFAs) and must be supplied by the diet.

The n-6 and n-3 series of fatty acids includes polyunsaturated fatty acids, or PUFAs, which are important components of animal and plant membranes and are precursors for prostaglandins and other eicosanoids. PUFAs are created though a series of reactions involving the elongation and desaturation of linoleic acid and α-linolenic acid. Linoleic acid is the precursor for the essential long-chain n-6 PUFA, arachidonic acid (AA).

Linoleic Acid (18:2n-6) ⇒ Arachidonic Acid (20:4n-6)

Linoleic acid is found in most vegetable oils, including corn, sunflower seed, safflower, cottonseed, soybean, and sesame oils. Arachidonic acid is a key precursor of several classes of signal molecules, including prostaglandins, prostacyclins, thromboxanes, and leukotrienes.[23] These four distinct groups of pharmacologically active compounds are called eicosanoids because they contain 20 carbon atoms. The inflammation response, vasoconstriction, platelet aggregation and immune response are just a few of the roles performed by eicosanoids. Desirable levels of arachidonic acid will promote a balanced production of eicosanoids and result in the body's appropriate response to injury or infection. However, in large amounts eicosanoids can induce a proaggregatory, prothrombic response with increased blood viscosity, vasospasm, and vasoconstriction.[20] These conditions can promote numerous health problems and diseases.

α-Linolenic acid is the precursor for essential long-chained n-3 PUFA, eicosapentanoic acid (EPA), and docosahexanoic acid (DHA).

α–Linolenic Acid (18:3n-3) ⇒ Eicosapentanoic Acid (20:5n-3) ⇒ Docosahexanoic Acid (22:6n-3)

α–Linolenic acid is present as a component of the chloroplast lipids in green leafy vegetables. Other sources of α-linolenic acid include flaxseed, soybeans, rapeseed, and walnuts. In addition, both eicosapentanoic acid and docosahexanoic acid can be provided directly by a diet high in fatty fish and fish oils. Fish consume marine phytoplankton, which results in high levels of EPA and DHA in the fish oils. As a general rule, cold water and marine fish contain more n-3 PUFA than warm water and freshwater fish.[6]

Eicosapentanoic acid and docosahexanoic acid can reduce eicosanoid production because n-3 and n-6 fatty acids compete for the same enzymes, Δ-6 desaturase and Δ-4 desaturase.[19] These enzymes display a higher affinity for the most unsaturated substrate and therefore, if present in the diet, will choose the n-3 fatty acid pathway (Fig. 4.1).

Eicosapentanoic acid and docosahexanoic acid promote effects that are hypolipidemic, antithrombic,[9,10,17] vasodilatory,[29] and anti-inflamatory.[20] Based on these benefits, n-3 fatty acids are shown to be preventative in heart disease, hypertension, adult onset diabetes, rheumatoid arthritis, chronic obstructive pulmonary disease, ulcerative colitis, and

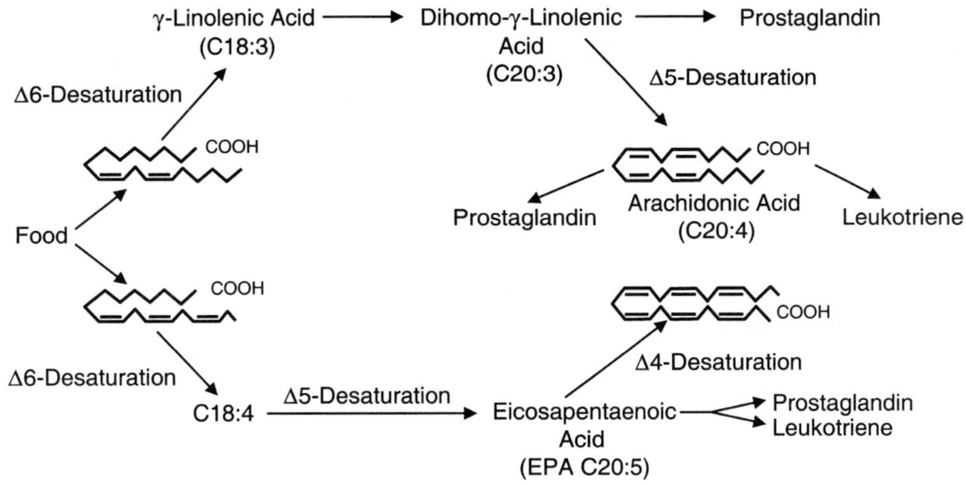

Figure 4.1. Metabolic pathways of n-6 and n-3 fatty acids. Modified from Reference 1.

Crohn's disease.[20] n-3 Fatty acids are also essential in the functional development of the retina and occipital cortex of the human fetus.[25] n-3 PUFAs have also recently been shown to display antiarrhythmic and anticonvulsant effects in animals and humans.[10]

Current and Recommended Dietary Intake of Essential Fatty Acids

Simopoulos[19] recommended, based on current knowledge of Paleolithic nutrition, a diet rich in wild game meats, plants, and nuts, all of which are high in α-linolenic acid. The ratio of n-6 to n-3 fatty acids was estimated to be 1–2:1, and the diet contained much lower levels of saturated fatty acids.[19] Today the ratio of n-6 to n-3 fatty acids is 20-30:1. This is due to several factors, such as reduced fish consumption and reduced levels of n-3 fatty acids in meat and eggs due to the formulation of animal feed high in n-6 fatty acids. In addition, the substitution of vegetable oils for saturated fatty acids in order to lower serum cholesterol levels has contributed enormously to the high dietary intake of n-6 fatty acids.[19] Modern cultivated plants contain lower levels of n-3 fatty acids than wild plants. Intake of n-3 fatty acids is estimated at 1.6 g/day of which 1.4 g is from α-linolenic acid and 0.1–0.2 g from EPA and DHA combined.

Currently, the United States does not have a recommended dietary allowance for essential fatty acids. An international scientific working group has estimated an adequate intake (AI) for both n-6 and n-3 fatty acids (Table 4.1).[22] The adequate intake of linoleic acid for adults on a 2,000 kcal diet is 4.44–6.67 g/day or 2–3 percent of energy. The adequate intake of α-linolenic acid is 2.22 g/day or 1 percent of energy.[22]

Table 4.1. Adequate intake (AI) of fatty acids for adults

Fatty acid	2,000 kcal diet (g/d)	Percentage of energy
LA	4.44	2.0
(Upper limit)	6.67	3.0
α–LNA	2.22	1.0
DHA + EPA	0.65	0.3
DHA to be at least	0.22	0.1
EPA to be at least	0.22	0.1
Trans-FA		
(Upper limit)	2.00	1.0
SAT		
(Upper limit)	—	<8.0
MONO	—	—

Source. Reference 19, 22.
Note. LA = linoleic acid, α-LNA = α-linolenic acid, DHA = docosahexanoic acid, EPA = eicosapentanoic acid, trans-FA = transfatty acid, SAT = saturated, and MONO = monounsaturated.

Specialty Eggs: Development of n-3 Fatty Acid–Enriched Chicken Eggs

The composition of the chicken egg yolk is highly sensitive to manipulation of the chicken's diet.[8] Studies as early as 1966–1967 showed that the degree of fatty acid composition in the egg yolk could be easily modified by the addition of various lipids to hen feed.[3,14] Several factors in the egg laying process determine the lipid content of the egg yolk: the incorporation of the lipid component of the diet, de novo lipogenesis, and the feedback inhibition of the dietary long-chain PUFA.[18]

Hen eggs produced under completely natural conditions, called Greek eggs, have been used as a composition guide for the development of n-3 fatty acid–enriched eggs (Table 4.2).[21] A typical supermarket egg has the ratio of n-6/n-3 fatty acids of 19.9:1, but the ratio of a Greek egg produced by a free-ranging chicken is 1.3:1. A hen fed with flax-flour–enriched feed produces an n-3–enriched specialty egg with the n-6/n-3 ratio of 1.6:1.[21]

In recent years, many studies have looked at finding the best formulation of hen feed that effectively raises the yolk's n-3 fatty acid content. A 1997 study by Van Elswyk[27] looked at the effects of various feed supplements—fish oil, flaxseed, or marine algae—on yolk lipid content and egg taste. Fish oil, rich in both EPA and DHA, was very effective in raising the n-3 PUFA content of the egg yolk at dietary levels of 15–30 g/kg, but it imparted an undesirable flavor to the egg. Ground flaxseed influenced the n-3 fatty acid content only at dietary levels 150 g/kg. The marine algae proved to be very efficient in raising the n-3 content of the egg yolk and provided naturally occurring carotenoids to the yolk, which enhanced the egg's oxidative stability.[27]

Table 4.2. Fatty acid levels (mg/g/yolk) in chicken egg yolks

Fatty acid	Greek egg	Supermarket egg
Saturates		
14:0	1.1	0.7
15:0	—	0.1
16:0	77.6	56.7
17:0	0.7	0.3
18:0	21.3	22.9
Total	100.7	80.7
Monounsaturates		
16:1n-7	21.7	4.7
18:1	120.5	110.0
20:1n-9	0.6	0.7
24:1n-9	—	—
Total	142.8	115.4
n-6 Polyunsaturates		
18:2n-6	16.0	26.1
18:3n-6	—	0.3
20:2n-6	0.2	0.4
20:3n-6	0.5	0.5
20:4n-6	5.4	5.0
22:4n-6	0.7	0.4
22:5n-6	0.3	1.2
Total	23.1	33.9
n-3 Polyunsaturates		
18:3n-3	6.9	0.5
20:3n-3	0.2	—
20:5n-3	1.2	—
22:5n-3	2.8	0.1
22:6n-3	6.6	1.1
Total	17.7	1.7
P:S	0.4	0.4
M:S	1.4	1.4
n-6:n-3 ratio	1.3	19.9

Source: Reference 20.

More recently, other nutrients have been added to hen feed to enrich the n-3 fatty acid eggs. A 2000 study by Meluzzi et al.[13] looked at the effects of enriching hen feed with vitamin E in the form of dl-α-tocopheryl acetate. Vitamin E and other antioxidants can prevent lipid oxidation, which was found to be a problem in eggs high in n-3 fatty acids produced from flaxseed-enriched feed.[16] Meluzzi et al. found that after 28 days of storage, the n-3 fatty acid, vitamin E–enriched eggs contained the same amount of vitamin E as on the first day. This suggests that the vitamin was not used to prevent lipid oxidation in the yolk. However, each egg supplied 100 to 200 mg/day of vitamin E, which helps to meet the Recommended Dietary Allowance.[13] Sim[18] found that incorporating vitamin E into hen feed helped reduce and stabilize off-flavor, volatile compounds, cholesterol oxidation products, and tetrabutylammonium (TBA) -reacting substances. Other studies have researched eggs that are enriched with multiple nutrients including DHA, vitamin E, lutein, and selenium.[24]

The Effects of n-3 Fatty Acid Specialty Eggs in Human Clinical Trials

Human clinical trials have helped to shed light on the effects of regular consumption of n-3–enriched eggs on serum cholesterol levels. Ferrier et al.[7] studied the influence on human serum lipids of eating four n-3–enriched eggs a day for 14 days. Within the group of 28 normolipidemic subjects, there were significant increases in DHA and total n-3 PUFAs in the blood platelet phospholipids. The ratio of n-6 to n-3 fatty acids in the platelets' phospholipids was significantly decreased. No significant changes were observed in total cholesterol, HDL (high-density lipoprotein), or triglyceride concentrations. A study by Farrell[6] evaluated changes in body weight, blood pressure, plasma lipid levels, and plasma n-3 PUFA levels. After consuming one n-3–enriched egg/day for 24 weeks, subjects had no significant changes in body weight, blood pressure, and plasma lipid levels. Between the control group and the n-3–enriched egg group, there was a significant increase of plasma EPA, DHA, and total n-3 PUFAs. The plasma ratio of n-6 to n-3 PUFAs was reduced from 12.1:1 to 6.5–7.7:1.[6]

Lewis et al.[11] looked at the effects of incorporating two n-3–enriched eggs a day into the low-fat diet of hyperlipidemic subjects. The study ran for 6 weeks. Of the 25 subjects, 2 responded with increased total serum cholesterol. The remaining subjects had no effects on their total cholesterol levels. As a group there was a 16 percent decrease in serum triglyceride levels when n-3–enriched eggs were consumed. This study suggests that, for the majority of the population, regular consumption of n-3–enriched eggs will not negatively alter blood lipid patterns. There is, however, a small subset of the hyperlipidemic population whose total and LDL (low-density lipoprotein) -cholesterol levels will increase with consumption of any regular or n-3–enriched egg.[11]

Conclusion

Development of n-3–enriched eggs appears to be a positive step toward promoting increased dietary intake of n-3 fatty acids in the general population. These eggs are enriched naturally, by supplementing hens' feed with fish oil, flaxseed, linseed oil, or marine algae. The addition of two n-3–enriched eggs per day to a low-fat diet can provide 1.4 g/day of n-3 PUFA.[11] This is approximately 50 percent of the proposed adequate intake of 2.22 g/day of α-linolenic acid for adults.[22] An increase of α-linolenic acid, EPA, and DHA can help to balance the gross imbalance of n-6 to n-3 fatty acids in the Western diet. Eicosapentanoic acid and docosahexanoic acids have been shown to play an important role in reducing blood pressure and viscosity, platelet aggregation, cardiac arrhythmia, and plasma triglycerides and are important to cardiac and immune health.[13] The list of benefits from increased dietary n-3 fatty acids includes the prevention and possible treatment of coronary heart disease, type II diabetes, rheumatoid arthritis, Crohn's disease, and chronic obstructive pulmonary disease.

Based on human clinical trials, n-3 fatty acid–enriched eggs can be a healthful addition to a low-fat diet without adverse effects on most people's serum cholesterol. n-3 Fatty acid–enriched eggs should be eaten in addition to other n-3 fatty acid–rich foods such as fish, leafy green vegetables, and selected vegetable oils in order to meet the suggested adequate intake of α-linolenic acid, EPA, and DHA. Other nutrients such as vitamin E, beta-carotene, selenium, and lutein are also being incorporated into these enriched eggs. n-3 Fatty acid–enriched eggs are currently available at most supermarkets and therefore are a convenient and beneficial food.

References

1. Abril, R., and Barclay, W. Production of docosahexanoic acid-enriched poultry eggs and meat, using algae-based feed ingredient. World Rev Nutr Diet 1998;83:77–88.
2. Baucells, M.D., Crespo, N., Barroeta, A.C., Lopez-Ferrer, S., and Grashorn, M.A. Incorporation of different polyunsaturated fatty acids into eggs. Poult Sci 1999;79:51–59.
3. Born, F. ω-3 Products: from research to retail. World Rev Nutr Diet 1998;83:166–75.
4. Cherian, G., and Sim, J.S. Changes in the breast milk fatty acids and plasma lipids of nursing mothers following consumption of n-3 polyunsaturated fatty acids enriched eggs. Nutrition 1996;12:8–12.
5. Eritsland, J. Safety considerations of polyunsaturated fatty acids. Am J Clin Nutr 2000;71:197S–201S.
6. Farrell, D.J. Enrichment of hen eggs with n-3 long chain fatty acids and evaluation of enriched eggs in humans. Am J Clin Nutr 1998;68:538–44.
7. Ferrier, L., Caston, L., Leeson, S., Squire, J., Weaver, B., and Holub, B. α-Linolenic acid and docosahexanoic acid enriched eggs from hen fed flaxseed: influence on blood lipids and platelet phospholipid fatty acids in humans. Am J Clin Nutr 1995;62:81–86.
8. Juneja, L.R. In Egg Yolk Lipids in Hen Eggs, Yamamoto, T., Juneja, L.R., Hatta, H., and Kim, M., eds. New York: CRC Press, 1997.
9. Leaf, A., and Kang, J.X. ω-3 Fatty acids and cardiovascular disease. World Rev Nutr Diet 1998;83:24–37.
10. Leaf, A., Kang, J.X., Xiao, Y.F., Billman, G., and Voskuyl, R. The antiarrhythmic and anticonvulsant effects of dietary n-3 fatty acids. J Membrane Biol 1999;172:1–11.
11. Lewis, N., Schalch, K., and Scheideler, S. Serum lipid response to n-3 fatty acid enriched eggs in persons with hypercholesterolemia. J Am Diet Assoc 2000;100:363–67.
12. Lewis, N., Seburg, S., and Flanagan, L. Enriched eggs as a source of n-3 polyunsaturated fatty acids for humans. Poult Sci 2000;79:971–74.
13. Meluzzi, A., Sirri, F., Manfreda, G., Tallarico, N., and Franchini, A. Effects of dietary vitamin E on the quality of table eggs enriched with n-3 long chain fatty acids. Poult Sci 2000;79:539–45.
14. Michella, S., and Slaugh, B. Producing and marketing a specialty egg. Poult Sci 2000;79:975–76.
15. Rose, D., and Connolly, J. Omega-3 fatty acids as cancer chemopreventative agent. Pharmacol Thera 1999;83:217–44.

16. Scheideler, S.E., Froning, G., and Cuppett, S. Studies of consumer acceptance of high omega-3 fatty acid-enriched eggs. J Appl Poult Res 1997;6:137–46.
17. Schmidt, E.B., and Dyerberg, J. n-3 Fatty acids and coronary heart disease—the urgent need of clinical trials. Lipids 1999;34:S303–5.
18. Sim, J. Designer eggs and their nutritional and functional significance. World Rev Nutr Diet 1998;83:89–101.
19. Simopoulos, A.P. Omega-3 fatty acids in health and disease and in growth and development. Am J Clin Nutr 1991;54:438–63.
20. Simopoulos, A.P. Essential fatty acids in health and chronic disease. Am J Clin Nutr 1999;70:560S–69S.
21. Simopoulos, A.P. New products from agri-food industry: the return of n-3 fatty acids into the food supply. Lipids 1999;34:S297–S301.
22. Simopoulos, A.P. Human requirements for n-3 polyunsaturated fatty acids. Poult Sci 2000;79:961–70.
23. Stryer, L. Biochemistry. 4th ed. New York: W.H. Freeman and Company, 1995, pp. 624–27.
24. Surai, P.F., A. MacPherson, B.K. Speake, and N.H.C. Sparks. Designer egg evaluation in controlled trial. Eur J Clin Nutr 2000;54:298–305.
25. Uauy, R., P. Peirano, D. Hoffman, P. Mena, D. Birch, and E. Birch. Role of essential fatty acids in the function and developing nervous system. Lipids 1996;31:S167–S176.
26. Valk, E.E.J. and G. Hornstra. Relationship between vitamin E requirement and polyunsaturated fatty acid intake in man: a review. Int J Vitam Nutr Res 2000;70:31–42.
27. Van Elswyk, M. Comparison of n-3 fatty acids sources in laying hen rations for improvement of whole egg nutritional quality: a review. Br J Nutr 1997;78:S61–S69.
28. Van Elswyk, M.K., S.D. Hatch, G.G. Stella, P.K. Mayo, and K.S. Kubena. Poultry-based alternatives for enhancing the ω3 fatty acid content of American diets. World Rev Nutr Diet 1998;83:102–15.
29. Von Schacky, C., P. Angerer, W. Kothny, K. Theisen, and H. Mudra. The effects of dietary ω-3 fatty acids on coronary atherosclerosis: a randomized, double–blind, placebo-controlled trial. Ann Intern Med 1999;130:554–62.
30. Zeman, F.J. Clinical Nutrition and Dietetics. 2nd ed. New York: Macmillan Publishing Company, 1991, pp. 351–52.

5

Vitamin E Enrichment of Chicken Eggs

Zeina Makhoul

Introduction

Eggs have long been an important food to humans and remain a popular food throughout the world. Eggs are nutritious. Although they contain 74 percent water, they are such a rich source of high-quality proteins that nutritionists often use them as a standard for measuring the quality of other proteins. Eggs are also an important source of unsaturated fatty acids (mainly oleic), iron, phosphorus, trace minerals, fat-soluble vitamins A, E, and K, and B vitamins.[1]

Eggs provide a unique, well-balanced source of nutrients for persons of all ages. Hen eggs contain many essential nutrients for chick embryo development and are considered an excellent food for humans. However, when considering human nutrition, it has been known for some time that there are several shortcomings associated with eggs. For example, eggs are a poor source of calcium (24 mg) and vitamin C (0 mg), and most importantly they have a very high cholesterol concentration (213 mg).[2]

Increasing Vitamin Content of Eggs

Because of the importance of eggs as a staple of the diet, attempts were made to manipulate the nutrient composition of eggs by changing hens' diets. These manipulations were reviewed by Naber in 1979.[3] Little or no variation was shown when amino acids, total proteins, carbohydrates, or minerals were changed in the diet, whereas fatty acids and vitamins, especially fat-soluble ones, showed a positive or marked influence on the egg content of these nutrients.

Fat-soluble vitamins are transferred from the hen's diet to the egg with some facility. The liver plays an important role in the uptake of nutrients and their deposition in egg yolk. High liver storage levels of a nutrient increase the egg content of this nutrient. According to Naber,[3] huge amounts of data are available about vitamins A, D, and B_{12} manipulation of chicken eggs, but insufficient data were found to characterize the relation between dietary concentration and egg content of vitamin E.

Increasing n-3 PUFA Content of Eggs

As mentioned before, the high cholesterol content of eggs posed a problem for the egg industry. Manipulation of eggs' cholesterol content failed to show any significant results. Instead, efforts were focused on increasing the polyunsaturated fatty acid (PUFA) content of eggs, which is easily changed by dietary manipulation of the laying hen. Attention given to modifying the fatty acid composition of eggs has recently focused on the elevation of omega-3 or n-3 fatty acids with the intention of making these products more favorable for human consumption.[4]

However, PUFAs are more prone to oxidation because of their double bonds, leading to the development of off-flavors, off-odors, and lower consumer acceptability. These oxidative phenomena can be prevented or limited by enriching the eggs with some active antioxidant such as vitamin E. Because of the antioxidant function of tocopherols as free radical scavengers, there is a greater awareness of tocopherols as having health benefits for preventing cancer, coronary heart disease, and inflammation. Thus, incorporating tocopherols into chicken eggs would increase oxidative stability and also contribute to meeting human vitamin E requirements.

This chapter presents studies and research done on vitamin E enrichment of eggs, especially n-3–modified ones, the difference in the transfer efficiency of tocopherol stereoisomers, and the benefits and effect of this enrichment on quality and sensory characteristics of table eggs.

Fat Metabolism in Chickens

Animals are unable to synthesize tocopherols and are dependent on dietary sources.[5] In avian populations, dietary supplementation of α-tocopherol has been reported to increase the α-tocopherol content of chicken eggs. Unlike mammals, chickens have a rudimentary lymphatic system. Thus, chylomicrons are absorbed directly into the portal blood for transport to liver for further synthesis and tissue deposition, allowing direct exposure of the liver to dietary fat and fat-soluble vitamins. This feature allows the manipulation of lipid and tocopherol content of hen eggs by dietary means.

The Rationale behind Designer Eggs

Many studies were done on improving the nutritional and cardioprotective properties of eggs via maternal diet manipulation with monounsaturated fatty acids (MUFAs) and PUFAs.[6] Recent efforts are aimed at increasing antioxidant vitamins. Eggs contain low levels of natural antioxidants; therefore, altering the PUFA composition of eggs may enhance susceptibility to lipid oxidation, resulting in lower quality, and may indicate a need for antioxidants. The main function of vitamin E is to protect susceptible cellular structures, especially PUFAs in cell membranes, against damage from oxygen-free radicals. Foods rich in vitamin E are from plant origins like seed oils, vegetables, and whole grains. Most animal products are poor sources of this vitamin.[6]

Tocopherol Contents

Most of the studies done about increasing the vitamin E content of eggs used the same chicken breed: Single Comb White Leghorn laying hens. All of them used vitamin E in addition to PUFA and MUFA supplementation. Furthermore, they all showed an increase of vitamin E concentration in eggs, egg yolk particularly.

This was supported by a study done by Qi and Sim[4] on 240 laying hens. The birds were fed an n-3 fatty acid–modified diet consisting of flaxseed and menhaden oil, with a natural tocopherol (TOC) mixture at 0, 200, 400, and 800 mg/kg for a period of 7 weeks. Eggs were collected from the four experimental groups and were analyzed for TOC content. The TOC contents of egg yolks increased linearly with increasing levels of dietary TOC up to 8 days of feeding, after which there was no apparent increase in the egg yolk TOC contents.

The largest study was done by Cherian et al.[5,7] using 480 laying hens. The chickens were fed diets based on wheat and soybean meal with added oils at 3.5 percent or oils plus mixed TOC. The composition of the dietary oils consisted of menhaden, palm, flax, or sunflower oils. The study's objective was to examine the effect of maternal dietary fat, varying in n-6 and n-3 fatty acids with or without added TOC, on the fatty acid and TOC status of chicks,[7] in addition to oxidative stability (discussed later) of chicken tissues.[5] After chickens were fed for 28 days, eggs and bird tissues were obtained for analysis. Results from the study indicate, like previous studies, that dietary oils and TOC produce a marked effect on the fatty acid composition and TOC content of eggs and hatched chick tissues.

The most recent study done on vitamin E–modified eggs is that of Meluzzi et al.[8] However, they used a different hen breed. Their study consisted of 192 Hy-Line Brown hens. They fed their birds with either lard or fish oil and four doses of dl-α-tocopheryl acetate (0, 50, 100, and 200 ppm). They reported that the amount of vitamin in the yolk was strictly related to the amount of α-TOC in the diet and increased linearly as dietary dl-α-tocopheryl acetate increased. It increased from the control level of 90.93 μg/g to 313.84 μg/g of yolk when 200 ppm was added to the hen's diet.

Tocopherol Composition

Up to now, studies on TOC enrichment of eggs have mainly focused on α-TOC. There is not enough consideration given to γ- and δ-TOC, which often exist in great quantities in natural sources and have higher oxidative activities in vitro than α-TOC.

In the Qi and Sim study,[4] different concentrations of TOC stereoisomers (α-, μ-, and δ-TOC) were found in the egg yolk (Fig. 5.1). The different TOC isomers were transferred to the eggs through diet. The TOC mixture used in this study consisted of 10 percent α-TOC, 60 percent γ-TOC, and 30 percent δ-TOC. Increasing the TOC supplementation in the diet (from 200 to 800 mg/kg) caused dietary γ- and δ-TOC increases, while dietary α-TOC decreased. However, egg yolk α-TOC accounted for half of the total content of eggs (Fig 5.2). So α-TOC had a higher efficiency of dietary transfer into eggs than γ- and

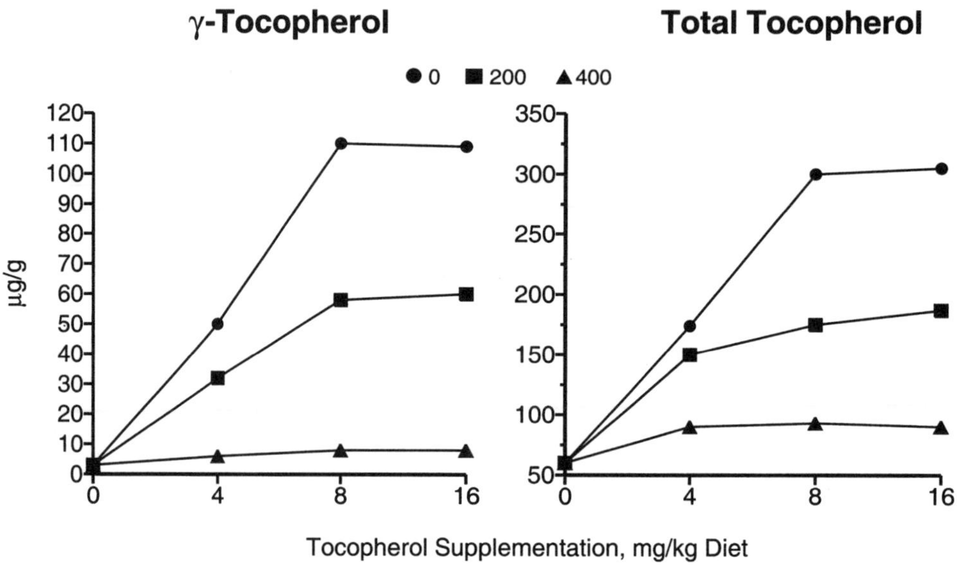

Figure 5.1. Tocopherol accumulation in egg yolks with time at different levels of tocopherol supplementation. Modified from Reference 4.

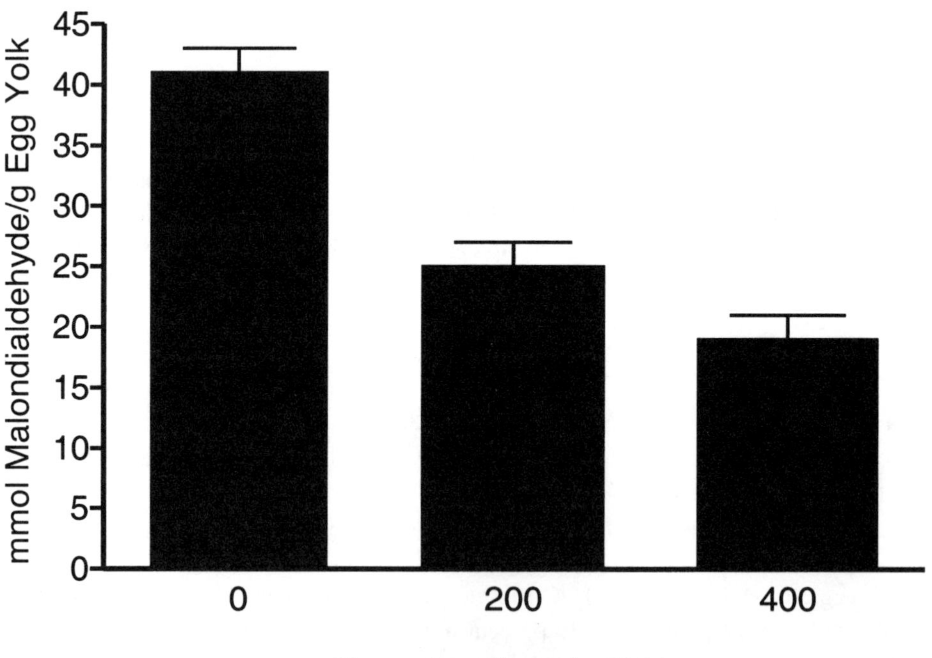

Figure 5.2. Comparison of tocopherol composition of diets and eggs. Modified from Reference 4.

δ-TOC. Nevertheless, eggs could also be enriched by γ- and δ-TOC dietary supplementation. Their higher antioxidative activity in vitro compared with that of α-TOC makes their enrichment in n-3 fatty acid–modified eggs more meaningful.

In their study, Piironen et al.[9] found that the transfer efficiencies of α-TOC stereoisomers are proportional to their biological activity. That is, the higher the biological activity, the more efficient the dietary transfer to eggs. This study examined the transfer of different stereoisomers of the α-TOC from feed to egg by comparing their stereoisomeric composition. *All-rac*-α-Tocopheryl acetate is the most common vitamin E preparation used in supplement feeds. This synthetic product is a mixture of eight isomers, which have been shown to have different biological activities. Acetate of the only naturally occurring isomer, α-TOC, has the highest activity. If researchers did not account for the presence of other stereoisomers, it would be possible that vitamin E activity would be overestimated to a certain extent. The actual activity of eggs was estimated to be about 80 percent of the value obtained when all TOC is determined as α-TOC.

Many other studies supported the same results as Piironen et al.[9] and Qi and Sim's[4] work. Cherian et al.[5,7] explained the preferential retention of α-TOC over other tocopherols in hens. They suggested that, in the mammalian system, the presence of a specific α-TOC–binding protein in the liver results in the preferential retention of γ-TOC and its subsequent release in very low-density lipoproteins (VLDLs).[5] Similarly, in chickens, the liver plays an important role in the metabolism of fat and fat-soluble vitamins. The tocopherols are transported via VLDLs to the egg yolk. Again, all of the TOC isomers were present in the egg yolk, which means that they were all transferred from diet to eggs, but in different amounts. The incorporation of different tocopherol isomers from feed to eggs in the order of magnitude was α-TOC > γ-TOC > δ-TOC.[2] δ-TOC was the least incorporated in the tissues despite its high dietary content in the study. This might be due to a selection process in favor of the other isomers or to factors that might have interfered with uptake of δ-TOC by the egg yolk.

Tocopherol with Other Antioxidants

Jiang et al.[10] studied the effect of α-TOC supplementation on chicken eggs to which other antioxidants like β-carotene were added. They supplemented the hens diet with β-carotene, dl-α-tocopheryl acetate, or their combination. In the TOC-supplemented group, Jiang et al. reported a linear increase from the control level of 144 μg/g to 477 μg/g of yolk when 400 mg dl-α-tocopheryl acetate/kg of diet was supplemented. β-Carotene and retinol levels also increased in the egg yolk of the experimental group, but the results were slight. However, the combined effects of α-TOC and β-carotene were more complex. Supplemental β-carotene markedly decreased the yolk deposition of α-TOC when the two compounds were fed together. This is due to the interference of one fat-soluble vitamin with the utilization of other fat-soluble vitamins. Therefore, increasing egg yolk β-carotene concentration in addition to vitamin E may not be economically feasible. The first reason is its low deposition efficiency relative to its supplementation cost. The second reason is its undesirable effect on reducing the retention of vitamin E by the egg yolk.

Tocopherol and Lipids

Yolk fat is of considerable importance in the nutrition of the developing chick embryo as a source of energy, essential fatty acids, and fat-soluble vitamins. The yolk of the average chicken egg contains around 6 g of lipid, mainly in the form of triglycerides (TGs) and phospholipids, and 0.54 α-tocopherol equivalents (α-TE) of vitamin E.[2] Over 80 percent of yolk lipids are absorbed by the embryo during the last week of incubation.[11] During their absorption, an increase of the "unsaturation" of yolk lipids occurs, leading to elevated amounts of longer-chain (LC) PUFAs. The high content of n-6 and n-3 fatty acids in the cell membrane increases the requirement for vitamin E in order to protect against peroxidative degradation. Noble et al. reported an investigation into the changing concentrations of α-TOC and the associated PUFA status of the liver during incubation.[11] α-TOC concentrations were low when the degree of unsaturation and risk of oxidation was high because of accumulation of LCPUFAs. This was at day 15 of incubation. The week just before hatching, α-TOC concentrations sharply increased in the liver, by which time PUFAs and the potential for oxidation were reduced significantly. Conversely, there was a decline in the concentration of α-TOC within the yolk content during the first 2 weeks of incubation, with a large reduction following this period. Thus, the need for antioxidant protection during late embryonic life may be attenuated by the LCPUFA composition of yolk lipids. At the particular time of high unsaturation, concentrations of α-TOC are minimal.[11]

Effect of Tocopherol on Fatty Acid Composition

Meluzzi et al.[8] investigated whether vitamin E addition is influenced by the type of lipid used. They used lard, fish oil, and different doses of vitamin E in order to study this effect. In contrast to lard, fish oils are very rich in PUFAs, especially n-3 fatty acids. The type of dietary lipid supplement did not significantly influence the vitamin E amounts. However, in all fish oil groups, a lower content of vitamin E was observed compared with that in the lard group. Meluzzi et al. suggested that high levels of dietary vitamin E associated with low levels of n-3 fatty acids reduce the total n-3 fatty acid deposition in the yolk, whereas high levels of dietary n-3 depress the vitamin E deposition.

Similar effects were shown in another study done by Cherian et al.[5] Results from this study show that dietary TOC produced a marked effect on the fatty acid composition of eggs. It appeared in the study that the longer-chain n-3 PUFAs in the n-3 fatty acid–modified eggs were protected from undergoing deterioration by TOC supplementation. The antioxidant potency of γ-TOC has been reported to be higher than that of α-TOC, as mentioned earlier.[7] Therefore, the lower level of γ-TOC in the liver and plasma of chicks that were fed a high-PUFA diet in vitro may suggest an increased usage of this TOC isomer due to the significantly higher levels of LCPUFAs in these tissues. These results may also suggest the need for TOC supplementation based on the PUFA content of diets.

Oxidative Stability

In all studies, chemical measurements of the oxidative stability of eggs were based on the thiobarbituric acid (TBA) of egg yolk (mg of MA per kg, where MA is malondialdehyde). Inclusion of TOC resulted in a significant reduction in the TBA values in eggs in the Cherian et al. study.[5] The TBA values of eggs fed on menhaden and flax diets were higher than those from palm and sunflower diets. The increased TBA values may be due to oxidative deterioration of LCPUFAs. This is often associated with a change in food flavors. A higher concentration of TOC-ameliorated lipid oxidation occurred in eggs of hens fed a high n-3 PUFA diet.

In the Qi and Sim study,[4] TBA values significantly decreased from 41.32 to 18.57 nmol of malondialdehyde/g of egg yolk. This indicates that the lipid stability of n-3 fatty acid–modified eggs could be improved by increasing their TOC content through dietary manipulation.

Also, Cherian et al.[7] reported that inclusion of the highest levels of TOC, which made antioxidants available to the birds, resulted in the lowest TBA values.

Effect of Tocopherol on Egg Parameters

According to Qi and Sim,[4] dietary TOC supplementation had no significant effect on egg production, feed consumption, and egg quality, which generally agrees with the work of Jiang et al.,[10] who reported no significant differences in egg production, egg yield, and egg weight when laying hens were fed a basal diet supplemented with 50, 100, 200, and 400 mg of dl-α-tocopheryl acetate/kg. However, they found that feed consumption decreased at the highest level of vitamin E supplementation.

This was also supported by the work of Meluzzi et al.,[8] who reported that performance of hens and egg parameters remained stable when birds were fed different types of lipid and levels of vitamin.

Effect of Tocopherol on Sensory Characteristics of Eggs

As for the organoleptic qualities of eggs, no significant differences were observed in taste and flavor measurements of scrambled egg samples among treatments.[4] At the highest level of TOC supplementation (800 mg/kg of diet), the egg flavor scored 3, where 1 is no off-flavor and 5 is strong off-flavor, while the taste scored 3.6, where 1 is dislike extremely and 5 is like extremely (Table 5.1).[4] These scores were better for lower TOC supplementation. So a very high vitamin E content in the diet may reduce the overall acceptability of eggs.

This observation is supported by a study done by Leeson et al.[12] on the organoleptic evaluation of eggs produced by hens fed flaxseed and vitamin E (Table 5.2). Aroma, flavor, and overall acceptability were unaffected by the level of both flax and vitamin E in the diet. Although there were significant differences found for off-flavor, these eggs were still considered acceptable to panelists. The highest scores for egg aroma, flavor, and over-

Table 5.1. Panel test results of scrambled eggs from laying hens fed different levels of tocopherols

	Tocopherol supplementation			
Parameter	0 mg/kg of diet	200 mg/kg of diet	400 mg/kg of diet	800 mg/kg of diet
Flavor[a]	2.49	2.73	2.55	3.04
Taste[b]	2.94	3.07	2.93	3.63

Note. Values expressed as mean of 20 observations and in a row have no significant difference ($P > 0.05$).
[a] Flavor score: 1, no off-flavor; 5, strong off-flavor.
[b] Taste score: 1, dislike extremely; 5, like extremely.
Modified from Reference 4.

Table 5.2. Sensory evaluation of eggs from hens fed flaxseed and vitamin E

Attribute	10 mg vitamin E No flaxseed	10 mg vitamin E 10% flaxseed	10 mg vitamin E 20% flaxseed	100 mg vitamin E 20% flaxseed
Egg aroma	5.17[a]	4.36[b]	4.83[a,b]	4.23[b]
Egg yolk flavor	5.15[a]	4.05[b]	3.85[b]	2.92c
Overall acceptability	5.32[a]	4.07[b]	3.96[b]	3.10c

Note. Hedonic scale used, with 7 = like very much and 1 = dislike very much.
[a–c] Mean values within a row with no common superscript differ significantly ($P < 0.05$).
Modified from Reference 4.

all acceptability were recorded for eggs from birds fed the lowest levels of flax and vitamin E, whereas the opposite scores were attributed to the highest levels. The experiment done in this study suggests that there may be a difference in overall acceptability due to high levels of vitamin E. This might be because vitamin E, if used at a very high concentration, may act as a pro-oxidant rather than an antioxidant. However, confirmation of this suggestion deserves further study.

Storage of Eggs

Eggs stored 28 days at room temperature showed a fatty acid composition similar to that observed in fresh eggs. However, in the stored eggs with the highest levels of vitamin E, the yolk contents of total n-3 were reduced significantly.[8] This reduction could be due to a pro-oxidant effect rather than an antioxidant effect of vitamin E when used at a very high concentration, as suggested by Leeson. [12] After 28 days of storage, the levels of vitamin E remained very close to those observed in fresh eggs, suggesting that the vitamin was not used to prevent lipid oxidation in the yolk.

Vitamin E is situated primarily in cell membranes, where it protects PUFAs from free-radical–induced oxidative damage. Such oxidative damage in the cell membranes may lead to the production of lipid peroxides. The increased presence of lipid peroxides can alter cellular functions and lead to the lysis of oxidized cell membranes. High levels of lipid peroxides in the yolk sac membrane of eggs stored over 2 weeks have been linked to lower hatchability. Reduced TOC content and higher TBA values have been reported in eggs stored over 10 days.[7]

Conclusion

The present consumer concerns about the nutritive value of foods have precipitated interest in the vitamin composition of eggs. The interest in modifying the level of vitamins in eggs now extends beyond production consideration to designing a high-quality food for consumption by health conscious humans.

All the information discussed in this chapter confirms that it is possible to produce designer eggs enriched with vitamin E, especially in n-3–modified chicken eggs, through dietary manipulation. The daily requirement for humans of n-3 fatty acids is estimated at approximately 100 to 200 mg. As for vitamin E, the human daily requirement depends on the amount of unsaturated fatty acids in the diet. However, it is recommended that about 10 mg/day be consumed. Thus, the consumption of one designer egg can match, according to the above recommendations, 50 percent to 100 percent of daily requirements. Therefore, the vitamin E–enriched egg is a very interesting food, as it is well-known that α-TOC is a free radical scavenger that has beneficial effects in preventing the onset of cancer and coronary heart disease.

This chapter provides insight into the forms of TOC that are most efficiently utilized and their role in maintenance of lipid stability in n-3 PUFA–modified chicken eggs. Further work explaining the mechanisms of absorption and metabolism of TOC in poultry will allow more efficient utilization of dietary fat and fat-soluble vitamins, which may help in providing a quality product acceptable to consumers.

References

1. Cook, F., and Briggs, G.M. Egg Science and Technology. 3rd ed. Westport, CT: Avi Publ., 1986, pp. 141–61.
2. Sizer, F., and Whitney, E. Nutrition: Concepts and controversies. 8th ed. Belmont, CA.: West/Wadsworth, 2000, Appendix A.
3. Naber, E.C. The effect of nutrition on the composition of eggs. Poult Sci 1979;58:518–28.
4. Qi, G-H., and Sim, J.S. Natural tocopherol enrichment and its effect in n-3 fatty acid modified chicken eggs. J Agric Food Chem 1998;46:1920–26.
5. Cherian, G., Wolfe, F.W., and Sim, J.S. Dietary oils with added tocopherols: effects on egg or tissue tocopherols, fatty acids, and oxidative stability. Poult Sci 1995;75:423–31.
6. Sim, J.I., Nakai, S., and Guenter, W. Egg Nutrition and Biotechnology. 1st ed. Wallingford, UK, New York: CABI Publ., 2000.
7. Cherian, G., and Sim, J.I. Egg yolk polyunsaturated fatty acids and vitamin E content alters the tocopherol status of hatched chicks. Poult Sci 1997;76:1753–59.
8. Meluzzi, A., Sirri, F., Manfreda, G., Tallario, N., and Franchini, A. Effects of dietary vitamin E on the quality of table eggs enriched with n-3 long-chain fatty acids. Poult Sci 2000;79:539–45.

9. Piironen, V.I., Liljeroos, A.I., and Koivistoinen, P.E. Transfer of α-tocopherol stereoisomers from feed to eggs. J Agric Food Chem 1991;39:99–101.
10. Jiang, Y.H., McGeachin, R.B., and Bailey, C.A. α-Tocopherol, β-carotene, and retinol enrichment of chicken eggs. Poult Sci 1994;73:1137–143.
11. Noble, R.C., Cocchi, M., and Bath, H.M. α-Tocopherol absorption and polyunsaturated fatty acid metabolism in the developing chick embryo. Br Poult Sci 1993;34:815–18.
12. Leeson, S., Caston, L., and MacLaurin, T. Organoleptic evaluation of eggs produced by laying hens fed diets containing graded levels of flaxseed and vitamin E. Poult Sci 1998;77:1436–40.

6

Reducing Infection in Infants with Egg Phospholipids

Yingying Liu
and Ronald R. Watson

Introduction

In infants, systemic infections resulting from bacterial, fungal, or viral agents are common because of their immature immune system and likelihood of exposure to infectious organisms on a daily basis.[1] One such infection, necrotizing enterocolitis (NEC), is an important cause of morbidity and mortality among preterm infants.[2] Presently, there is not a way to predict the onset of the disease or to prevent its occurrence. Some interventions to infection, including enhanced barrier function, immunoprotection, and bacteriostasis (antibiotics, low pH formula), are associated with problems such as poor availability, metabolic acidosis, or antibiotic resistance.[3,4] Some epidemiologic and experimental studies have established that addition of egg phospholipids (PLs) to formula feedings could reduce infant infection.[5,6]

Eggs have been recognized as an important food from the time primitive men first snatched them from the nests of wild birds. Today, eggs remain a popular food in all countries of the world, providing a unique, well-balanced source of nutrients for persons of all ages. They are a particularly rich source of high-quality protein and PLs. Their high nutrient content, low caloric value, and ease of digestibility make them valuable in many therapeutic diets. They help patients return to good health and maintain it.[7]

There are numerous reviews on the potential importance of including long-chain fatty acids such as arachidonic acid (AA) and docosahexanoic acid (DHA), which are the components of egg PLs, in the diets of preterm and term infants.[8,9] Based upon the existing literature, dietary egg PLs can confer a degree of control over viral infectivity in vivo. This may contribute to the role of PLs in boosting antigen-induced immune response in mammals. Egg PLs given as dietary supplements also show promise for the prevention or alleviation of syndromes related to membrane lipid insufficiencies or abnormalities.[10] This chapter examines the expected numbers of infections in infants, the components of egg PLs, and the evidence and mechanisms for reducing infection in infants fed formula with egg PLs.

Expected Infections in Infants

Every pediatrician is faced with the fact that some infants have more infections than others. The expected types of infection in infants include *viral* and *bacterial* infections. Acute respiratory tract infections (RTIs) are the most common viral infection in people, and mostly acute upper RTIs are common in infants and children.[11] Rhinoviruses, adenoviruses, influenza viruses, and parainfluenza viruses cause the greatest proportion of acute respiratory illness.[12] Newborn infants can be HIV-positive because of an HIV-infected mother.

For the infant or child who has abdominal complaints and diarrhea caused by bacteria, it is important to identify the water supply, a potential source of bacteria. Various combinations of inadequate tissue oxygenation, bacterial overgrowth, and enteral feeding with immaturity may cause the initial damage to intestinal mucosa that culminates in necrosis. For example, necrotizing enterocolitis (NEC) causes approximately 4,000 deaths per year and significant morbidity among U.S.-born preterm infants alone.[2]

Exposure and *nutrition* can exacerbate infections. An infant or child interacting with other children increases the risk of infection transmission. Additionally, many epidemiological and experimental studies have established that environmental tobacco smoke is harmful to people's health, especially infants and children.[13] Malnutrition, including vitamin or micronutrient or fatty acid, is associated with increased incidence of severity of infection, including respiratory infection.[14]

Infections are not uncommon in infants, because infants have immune systems that are maturing, and infants and children are often exposed to infectious organisms on a daily basis. However, frequency, chronicity, or severity of infection is often abnormal, which may be caused by immunodeficiency.

The Components of Egg PLs

Shell eggs consist of about 9.5 percent shell, 63 percent albumin, and 27.5 percent yolk. The albumin contains only 0.03 percent lipids, while the yolk is the main source of lipids in the eggs. The lipid content of the yolk from eggs of various strains of hens is between 32 and 36 percent. In a review,[7] Privett et al. found that the composition of yolk lipids is 65.5 percent triglyceride, 28.3 percent PLs, and 5.2 percent cholesterol while Rhode and Lea calculated the composition of yolk PLs as 73 percent phosphatidylcholine (PC), 15 percent phosphatidylethanolamine (PE), 5.8 percent lysophosphatidylcholine (LPC), 2.5 percent sphingomyelin (SPM), 2.1 percent lysophosphatidylethanolamine (LPE), 0.9 percent plasmalogen, and 0.6 percent inositol phospholipid (IP).[7]

The fatty acid composition of lipid fractions of yolk is presented in Table 6.1. It is of interest to note that the total amounts of palmitic and stearic acids in PLs are high, which are about 49 percent for lecithin and about 54 percent for cephalin. The fatty acid composition of PLs also includes oleic acid (18:2n-2), linoleic acid (18:2n-6, LA), arachidonate (20:4n-6, AA), and docosahexaenoate (22:6-3n, DHA).[7] For example, the amount

Table 6.1. Fatty acid composition of lipid fractions of yolk and dietary lipid

	Percentage of total fatty acids				
Fatty acid	Crude lipid	Triglyceride	Lecithin	Cephalin	Dietary lipid
16:0	23.5	22.5	37.0	21.6	14.0
16:1	3.8	7.3	0.6	trace	2.7
18:0	14.0	7.5	12.4	32.5	2.4
18:1	38.4	44.7	31.4	17.3	29.1
18:2	16.4	15.4	12.0	7.0	44.4
18:3	1.4	1.3	1.0	2.0	3.2
20:4	1.3	0.5	2.7	10.2	0.8
22:5	0.4	0.2	0.8	3.0	0.8
22:6	0.8	0.6	2.1	6.4	1.3

necessary to supply even the lowest amounts of AA and DHA in egg PLs will result in a formula with considerably more cholesterol than is usually present in human milk.[15] Some evidence exists that addition of these long-chain polyunsaturated fatty acids (LCPUFAs) to infant formulas may be beneficial with respect to reducing infection.

Evidence for Reducing Infection in Infants Fed Formula with Egg PLs

Formulas marketed in North America do not contain LCPUFAs. With few exceptions, formula feeding results in lower plasma cholesterol, particularly apo B–containing lipoproteins, and lower AA and DHA concentrations than breast feeding.[16,17] Some evidence also suggests that early nutrition may influence chronic disease, including coronary heart disease, in adult humans.[18] Fortunately, inclusion of egg PLs in the formula could increase plasma HDL (high-density lipoprotein) -cholesterol concentration and liver and bile PLs, AA, and DHA in the formula-fed piglet.[19] Much of the current interest with respect to AA and DHA in infant lipid nutrition has focused on the important role of AA and DHA in growth and brain and visual function.[16,17,20] Studies have also been done to demonstrate PL function in reducing infections in infants. Recent controlled clinical observations using a randomized and masked design in premature infants suggest that a formula containing egg PLs as a source of LCPUFAs (DHA and AA) may reduce the incidence of NEC. The control formula-fed infants (n = 85) had a 17.6 percent prevalence of proven NEC, whereas the PL (n = 34) formula-fed infants had only 2.9 percent. In a previous study this same investigator reported an insignificant association of LCPUFA supplementation and increased NEC incidence. Therefore, this researcher speculated that one or more of the components present in the egg PLs enhanced gut maturation. LCPUFAs, PLs, or choline could potentially mediate this protective response.[6] Small clinical trials to evaluate egg PLs in HIV-associated disease were conducted in the United States, Israel, and West Germany 10 years ago.[21,22,23] Although these trials have suffered inadequate design, the available data do indicate that daily ingestion of egg yolk PLs as part of a structured dietary regimen can benefit the quality of life for many people with AIDS or other symptomatologies. Laboratory data showed that red cell, white cell, and platelet counts tend to improve and counts of T_4/helper and T_8/suppressor cells may increase marginally. Lymphocyte mitogenic responses also seem to improve, and HIV activity is reduced. Clearly, egg PLs are not a cure for HIV-1 infection. However, properly prepared and administered, the egg PLs can have virustatic and immune-restorative effects.

The Possible Mechanism of Egg PLs to Reduce Infection in Infants

A good deal of evidence suggests that dietary egg yolk PLs can confer a degree of control over viral infectivity in vivo.[10] The mechanism can be summarized in two points. (1) *Interference with viral envelope formation:* For example, herpes simplex virus (HSV), measles virus, and influenza virus are all enveloped viruses that can occur in infants. Depletion of the cholesterol of the virus envelope by incubation with egg lecithin micelles or with serum lipoprotein enriched with PLs also results in disruption of the envelope and loss of viral infectivity. (2) *Protection or restoration of transmembrane signaling functions in host cells:* Egg PL-containing formulas can provide animal-source PE and smaller amounts of other PLs, including phosphatidylinositol (PI) and phosphatidylserine (PS) to the inner leaflet of the plasma membrane, mainly to maintain the membrane's signal transduction function.

Activation of immune cells by egg PL-containing formula may be another way to reduce viral or bacterial infections.[10] It has been established that the maintenance of immune cells in culture requires exogenous fatty acids. PLs have a significant role in boosting antigen-induced immune responses in mammals. Fatty acids of PLs can be metabolized to eicosanoids (prostaglandins, thromboxanes, and leukotrienes), cytokines (diacylglycerol, platelet-activating factor, phosphatidic acid, and lipoxins), and other hormonelike factors (Fig. 6.1).[24] The lipoxygenated products seem to be mediators in the inflammatory process and immunoregulation.

Conclusion

Egg PLs as a dietary supplement have diverse potential application and an enviable ratio of benefit to risk. The components of egg PLs include AA, DHA, and choline. Their metabolic products may play an important role in membrane integrity, functional modulation of the membrane, and activation of immune cells. This may possibly reduce the risk of infant infection. Recently, more researchers have shown interest in the important role of egg PLs in growth and nervous system and visual functions. However, research on the effects of egg PLs on infant infection is limited. The exact mechanism of how egg PLs reduce infection, the safe doses of egg PLs that can be added to the formula of infants, and

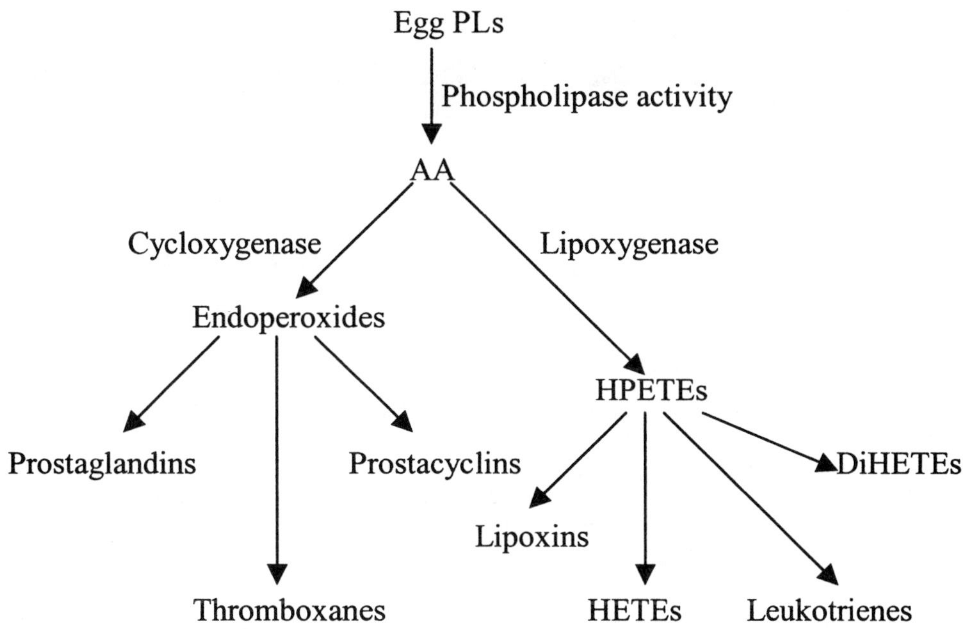

Figure 6.1. Major pathways of synthesis of eicosanoids from arachidonic acid. HPETE = hydroperoxyeicosatetranoic acid, HETE = hydroxyeicosatetranoic acid, and DiHETE = dihydroxyeicosapentanoic acid.

the role of other components of egg PLs are still poorly understood. Therefore, there is much that can be learned by researchers interested in infant infection and egg PL formula supplementation.

REFERENCES

1. Paul, M.E., and Shearer, W.T. The child who has recurrent infection. Immun Allergy Clin North Am 1999;19:423–36.
2. Brown, E.G., and Sweet, A.Y. 1990. Neonatal necrotizing enterocolitis. Pediatr Clin North Am 1982;29:1149–70.
3. Carrion, V., and Egan, E.A. Prevention of neonatal necrotizing enterocolitis. J Pediatr Gastroenteral Nutr 11:317–23.
4. Egan, E.A., Nelson, R.M., Mantilla, G., and Eitzman, D.V. Additional experience with routine use of oral kanamysin prophylaxis for necrotizing enterocolitis in infants under 1000 g. J Pediatr 1977;93:31–32.
5. Uauy, R.D., Fanaroff, A.A., Korones, S.B., and Phillips, E.A., Phillips, J.B., and Wright, L.L. Necrotizing enterocolitis in very low birth weight infants: biodemographic and clinical correlates. J Pediatr 1991;119:630–38.
6. Carlson, S.E., Montalto, M.B., Ponder, D.L., Weakman, S.H., and Korones, S.B. Lower incidence of necrotizing enterocolitis in infants fed a preterm formula with egg phospholipids. Pediatr Res 1998;44:491–98.

7. Stadelman, W.J., and Cotterill, O.J. Egg Science and Technology. New York: Food Products Press, 1990.
8. Decsi, T., and Koletzko, B. Polyunsaturated fatty acids in infant nutrition. Acta Paediatr Suppl 1994;83:31–37.
9. Hamosh, M., and Salem, N., Jr. Long-chain polyunsaturated fatty acids. Biol Neonate 1998;74:106–20.
10. Israel, H., and Giancarlo, P. Phospholipids: Biochemical, Pharmaceutical and Analytical Considerations. New York: Plenum Press, 1990.
11. Campbell, H. Acute respiratory infection: a global challenge. Arch Dis Child 1995;73:281–83.
12. Monto, A.S. Viral respiratory infections in the community: epidemiology, agents and interventions. Am J Med 1995;99:24S–27S.
13. Li, J.S., Peat, J.K., Xuan, W., and Beny, G. Meta-analysis on the association between environmental tobacco smoke (ETS) exposure and the prevalence of lower respiratory tract infection in early childhood. Pediatr Pulmonol 1999;27:5–13.
14. English, R.M., Badcock, J.C., Giay, T., Ngu, T., Waters, A.M., and Bennett, S.A. Effect of nutrition improvement project on morbidity from infectious diseases in preschool children in Vietnam: comparison with control commune. BMJ 1997;315:1122.
15. Heird, W.C. Biological effects and safety issues related to long–chain polyunsaturated fatty acids in infants. Lipids 1999;34:207–14.
16. Innis, S.M., Akrabawi, S.S., Diersen-Schade, D.A., Dobson, M.V., and Guy, D.G. Visual acuity and blood lipids in term infants fed human milk or formulae. Lipids 1997;32:63–72.
17. Auestad, N., Montalto, M.B., Hall, R.T., Fitzgerald, K.M., Wheeler, R.E., Connor, W.E., Neuringer, M., Connor, S.L., Taylor, J.A., and Hartmann, E.E. Visual acuity, erythrocyte fatty acid composition, and growth in term infants fed formulas with long chain polyunsaturated fatty acids for one year, Ross Pediatric Lipid Study. Pediatr Res 1997;41:1–10.
18. Barker, D.J.P. Fetal nutrition and cardiovascular disease in adult life. Lancet 1993;341:938–41.
19. Devlin, A.M., and Innis, S.M. Dietary phospholipid alters biliary lipid composition in formula-fed piglets. Lipids 1999;34:1313–18.
20. Innis, S.M. Essential fatty acids in growth and development. Prog Lipid Res 1991;30:39–103.
21. Goebel, F.D., and Bogner, J. Clinical findings after administration of lipids in AIDS—a pilot study. IVth Int Conf AIDS. Stockholm, Abstr. No.3531. 1988.
22. Skornick, Y., and Yust, I. Treatment of AIDS patient with AL 721. IVth Int Conf AIDS. Stockhom, Abstr. No. 3529. 1988.
23. Yust, I., Vardinon, N., Skornick, Y., Zakuth, V., Hasner, A., and Shinitzky, M. Reduction of circulating HIV antigen in sero-positive patients after treatment with AL 721. IVth Int Conf AIDS. Stockholm, Abstr. No. 3530. 1988.
24. Ziegler, E., and Filer, L. Present knowledge in nutrition. Washington, DC: ILSI Press, 1996.

7

Generation of Polyclonal Antibodies in the Egg Yolk

Max Gassmann

INTRODUCTION

Avian embryos and neonates acquire passive immunity by transfer of maternal antibodies from serum to egg yolk. Despite being classified as an IgG-like immunoglobulin, the structure of chicken egg yolk antibody (termed IgY) differs considerably from that of mammalian IgG. For example, while the molecular weight of mammalian IgG heavy chain is about 50 kDa, the one from chicken is 67–70 kDa.[1] Moreover, there are differences in the number of constant domains of the heavy chain (four in avian antibodies versus three in mammalian antibodies), in the number and nature of carbohydrate chains, and in the structure of the hinge region, which is more rigid in the chicken antibodies.[2] IgY antibodies do not cross-react with mammalian immunoglobulins, do not activate mammalian complement, and do not bind protein A or G. Although the last feature is often viewed as a disadvantage, it is easily overcome by using an intermediate mammalian antibody raised against IgY.[3] Moreover, a novel synthetic ligand mimicking protein A in the recognition of the immunoglobulin Fc portion was recently identified.[4] The specificity of this ligand was much broader than that of protein A since it efficiently bound both mammalian IgG and chicken IgY. Owing to the phylogenetic distance, conserved mammalian proteins are often more immunogenic in birds than in mammals.[5,6] Indeed, a successful production and application of IgY antibody against a highly conserved protein mannose-6-phosphate/insulinlike growth factor II receptor (M6P/IGFII-R) has recently been reported.[7] Compared with antibody production in rabbits, the IgY technology offers several advantages: (1) no bleeding but egg collection is required upon immunization, (2) IgY isolation is fast and simple, and (3) very low quantities of antigen are required to obtain high and long-lasting IgY titers in the yolk from immunized hens.[6]

This technique has been used to generate IgY antibodies against the α-subunit of the human hypoxia-inducible factor-1 (HIF-1). The adaptation to hypoxia involves the specific activation of oxygen-regulated genes such as erythropoietin, vascular endothelial growth factor, and transferrin (reviewed by Wenger and Gassmann).[11] Induction of these genes is mediated by HIF-1, a heterodimeric transcription factor composed of the two subunits HIF-1α and HIF-1β: while HIF-1α represents a newly detected protein, HIF-1β was found to be identical to the heterodimerization partner of the dioxin receptor/aryl hydrocarbon receptor (AhR), termed AhR nuclear translocator (ARNT). It has been shown that HIF-1β/ARNT is indispensable for HIF-1 DNA binding and transactivation function.[12,13] The observation that homozygous mice lacking HIF-1α die shortly after midgestation[14–16] indicates that HIF-1 is a nonredundant master regulator of oxygen homeostasis. Affinity purified anti-HIF-1α IgY antibodies enabled us to detect HIF-1α protein in electrophoretic mobility shift assays (EMSAs), immunoblots, and immunofluorescence experiments using hypoxic cells from different mammalian cell lines.

Material and Methods

Generation of Anti–HIF-1α IgY Antibodies

Antigen preparation and hen immunization were performed as described.[17] In brief, the PCR-amplified fragment of the human HIF-1α cDNA-spanning[18] amino acids 530 to 825 was overexpressed as a fusion protein with glutathione S-transferase. Following purification by Glutathione Sepharose 4B, the GST-HIF-1$\alpha_{530-825}$ antigen underwent electrophoresis in a preparative SDS polyacrylamide gel, and the corresponding band was excised and lyophilized. Approximately 60–80 µg antigen were resuspended in 500 µl PBS, emulsified with an equal volume of Freund's complete adjuvant, and injected into the pectoral muscle of hens at days 0, 14, and 28. Note that to further reduce animal suffering, biocompatible adjuvants different from Freund's complete adjuvant have been found to be considerably less harmful for animals, but almost as effective in inducing antibody titer in chickens.[19]

Rapid isolation of polyclonal chicken antibody from individual eggs that were collected daily was performed by a simple two-step procedure modified from an earlier protocol:[20] after separation from the egg white, the yolk was brought to 25 ml with sodium phosphate buffer (100 mM, pH 7.6) and mixed vigorously. Subsequently, chloroform (20 ml) was added, and the mixture was shaken until a semisolid phase was obtained. After centrifugation at 1,200 × g for 30 minutes, the supernatant was decanted and solid polyethylene glycol 6,000 was added to a final concentration of 12 percent (w/v). Following centrifugation at 15,700 × g for 10 minutes, the pellet was resuspended in 2 ml sodium phosphate buffer and stored at – 80°C. Of note, a number of methods exist for the fast and easy isolation of IgY from egg yolk.[21,22]

Affinity Purification of IgY Antibodies

Recombinant fusion protein (2.5 mg) containing the human HIF-1α C-terminus was coupled to 1 gram of reswollen cyanogen bromide-activated Sepharose 4B (Pharmacia) according to the manufacturer's instructions. After rinsing the column with 50 ml PBS, isolated IgY fractions from four eggs were pooled (8 ml), brought to 50 ml with PBS, and loaded overnight at 4°C. The column was washed with 50 ml PBS and bound IgY was eluted with 8.5 ml of elution buffer (0.15 M sodium chloride, 0.2 M glycine, pH 2.2). For immediate neutralization, the eluted fractions (2 ml) were poured into 15 ml tubes containing 0.8 ml of 1 M Tris-HCl buffer (pH 8.0). Prior to storage of the affinity purified IgY antibodies at −20°C, 0.1 mg/ml bovine serum albumin was added as carrier.[8]

Cell Culture

The human epithelioid carcinoma cell line HeLa, the African green monkey cell line COS-7, the mouse hepatoma cell line Hepa1, the porcine kidney cell line LLC-PK1, and the canine kidney cell line MDCK were cultured in incubators in which the oxygen partial pressure was either 140 mm Hg (20 percent O_2 v/v, normoxia) or 7 mm Hg (1 percent O_2 v/v, hypoxia). Routinely, cells at a density of approximately $1–2 \times 10^5$ cells/cm^2 were subjected to hypoxic induction for 4 hours.

EMSA and Immunoblot

Nuclear extracts from hypoxic and normoxic cells were isolated exactly as described.[23] EMSA analysis was performed using an erythropoietin gene-derived oligonucleotide containing the HIF-1 DNA-binding site.[23] For supershifts analysis, 1 µl of IgY antibody was added to the binding reaction. For immunoblot analysis, total cell lysates underwent electrophoresis through an SDS polyacrylamide gel and transferred to a nitrocellulose membrane using standard methodology. The membrane was blocked with 4 percent (w/v) instant nonfat milk powder and incubated for 2 hours with the affinity purified IgY antibody diluted in PBS containing 4 percent milk powder. Subsequently, the membranes were incubated with horseradish peroxidase–coupled rabbit anti–chicken antibodies (Promega, G1351) for 1 hour and developed using the Super Signal Chemiluminescent Substrate (Pierce).

Indirect Immunofluorescence Microscopy

Normoxic and hypoxic Hepa1 and COS-7 cells were fixed with 4 percent formaldehyde (pH 8.0) for 10 minutes at room temperature, washed three times with PBS, permeabilized with 0.5 percent Triton X-100 in PBS for 5 minutes and rinsed again with PBS. Unspecific binding was blocked by adding 10 percent fetal calf serum in PBS for 30 minutes. Cells were incubated with the affinity purified IgY antibody (diluted 1:10 in PBS) at 37°C for 1 hour IgY antibody was detected by using an FITC-conjugated rabbit anti–chicken antibody (Promega, G2691) at room temperature for 30 minutes. Following extensive washing in PBS and mounting in DABCO solution (Sigma), immunofluorescence was analyzed by confocal laser scanning microscopy.

Results and Discussion

Egg yolk antibodies from hens immunized with the human HIF-1α fusion protein were extracted from individual eggs. Based on its simplicity and rapidity, a modified chloroform-polyethylene glycol procedure was chosen that very efficiently enriched for chicken immunoglobulins. Using this optimized protocol, IgY was purified to better than 90 percent homogeneity (Fig. 7.1A). To test their specificity, it was determined whether IgY antibodies were capable of recognizing native HIF-1α protein in EMSAs using as probe an HIF-1 DNA-binding oligonucleotide derived from the erythropoietin gene. Following incubation of the probe with nuclear extracts from normoxic or hypoxic HeLa cells, the expected nonspecific, constitutive, and hypoxia-inducible factors were detected (Fig. 7.1B). Addition of the chicken polyclonal antibody partially abolished binding of the HIF-1 heterodimer to the HIF-1 DNA-binding site and partially supershifted the HIF-1 complex, whereas the constitutive and the nonspecific factors were not affected.

Immunoblot analysis using nuclear fractions from HeLa cells revealed the presence of specific IgY antibodies in eggs collected as early as 1 day after the last antigen injection (data not shown). Strong background signals in these experiments, however, forced us to affinity purify the IgY antibodies. Routinely, pooled polyethylene glycol fractions from four egg yolks yielded 14–16 ml affinity purified IgY that detected HIF-1α in nuclear extracts from hypoxic HeLa cells at a dilution as high as 1:1000 (Fig. 7.1C). It was next determined whether the IgY antibody was capable of recognizing HIF-1α protein present in cell lines from different mammals. To this end, human (HeLa), monkey (COS-7), swine (LLCPK), dog (MDCK), and mouse (Hepa1) cells were exposed to hypoxia (1 percent oxygen) for 4 hours. Immunoblot analysis using nuclear extracts derived from induced cells detected abundant HIF-1α protein in all mammalian cells tested (Fig. 7.1D).

To determine the subcellular localization of HIF-1α, Hepa1 and COS-7 cells were analyzed that were exposed to normoxia (20 percent oxygen) and hypoxia (1 percent oxygen) by indirect immunofluorescence and confocal laser scanning microscopy using the affinity purified IgY antibody. When grown in normoxic conditions, a weak signal was observed in both, in the cytoplasm and nuclei of the cells (Fig. 7.2). Hypoxic exposure for 4 hours resulted in a drastic increase of HIF-1α in the nucleus excluding nucleoli. Considering that the heterodimerization partner HIF-1α/ARNT is present in the nucleus, too, high levels of HIF-1α protein during hypoxia might be explained by increased stabilization of both HIF-1 subunits after heterodimerization. Using our IgY antibody as well as cell lines mutant for HIF-1α or HIF-1β/ARNT, we recently showed that HIF-1 accumulation in the nuclei of hypoxic cells was independent of the presence of HIF-1β/ARNT but that heterodimerization is required for stable association within the nuclear compartment.[3]

Despite its general applicability and advantages, the IgY technology is scarcely used so far. Because (1) chicken housing is inexpensive, (2) egg collection is nonstressful to the hens, (3) isolation and affinity purification of IgY antibodies is fast and simple, and (4) the applicability of IgY is widespread, immunization of hens represents an excellent alternative to generate polyclonal antibodies.[9,10]

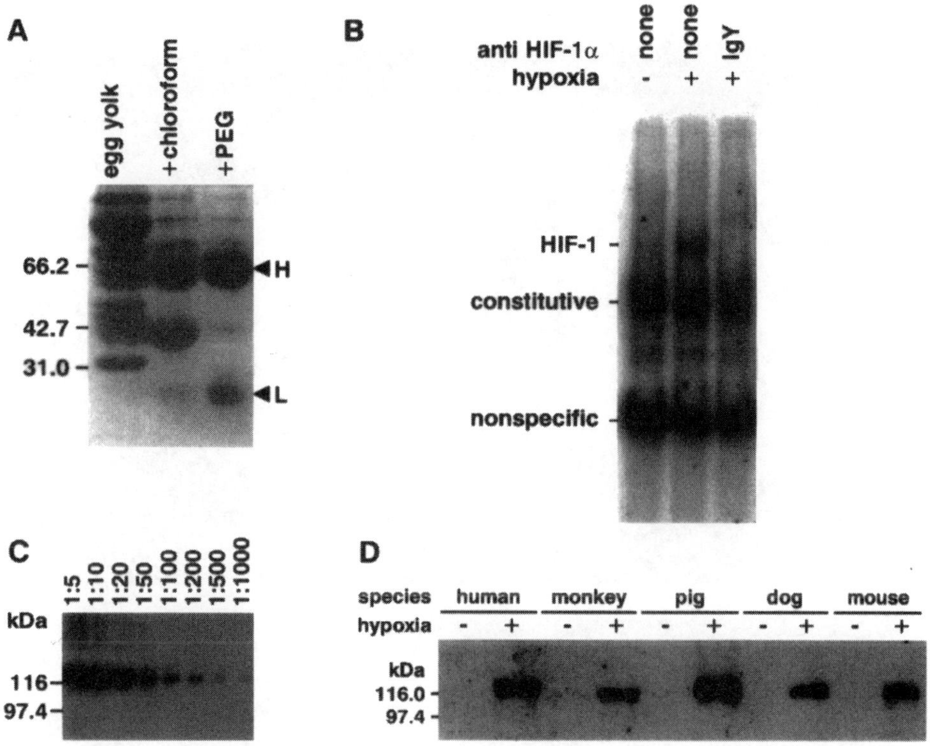

Figure 7.1. Characterization of anti-HIF-1α IgY antibody. (**A**) Electrophoretic separation of egg yolk IgY antibodies in a 10 percent SDS polyacrylamide gel. Egg yolk = crude yolk extract (30 μg protein), +chloroform = egg yolk supernatant after chloroform extraction (10 mg protein), and +PEG: chloroform-extracted egg yolk supernatant after precipitation with polyethylene glycol and resuspension in PBS (5 μg protein). H, L = heavy and light chain of chicken IgY. (**B**) Anti-HIF-1α IgY antibody recognizes native HIF-1α. Nuclear extracts (5 μg) from normoxic or hypoxic HeLa cells were analyzed by EMSA. The DNA-binding activity of the HIF-1 complex drastically decreased upon incubation with the chicken polyclonal anti-HIF-1α IgY antibody. (**C**) Immunoblot analysis using affinity purified anti-human HIF-1α IgY antibodies. Nuclear extracts (100 μg) from hypoxic HeLa cells were incubated with affinity purified IgY antibodies at the indicated dilutions. (**D**) The polyclonal IgY antibody recognizes HIF-1α from a variety of mammalian cells. Anti-HIF-1α IgY antibodies detected HIF-1α protein in extracts from human cervical carcinoma (HeLa), African green monkey kidney (COS-7), pig kidney (LLCPK1), dog kidney (MDCK), and mouse hepatoma (Hepal) cell lines. Total cell lysates (50 μg) were resolved by 7.5 percent SDS-PAGE, and immunoblots were analyzed with affinity purified IgY antibodies at a dilution of 1:100.

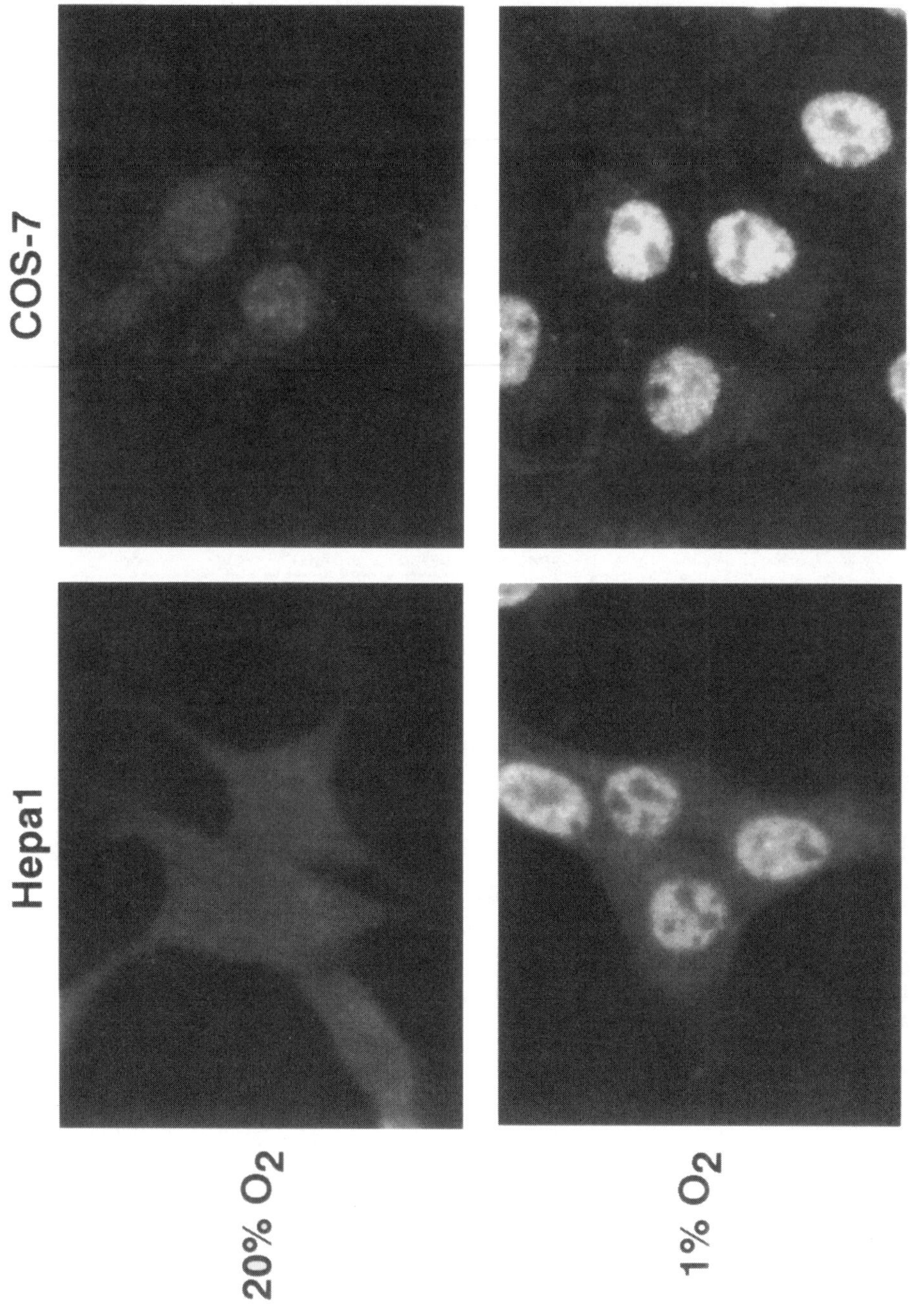

Figure 7.2. Analysis of HIF-1α expression in normoxic and hypoxic Hepal and COS-7 cells. Mouse Hepal and monkey COS-7 cells were cultured at normoxia or hypoxia (20 percent or 1 percent oxygen, respectively) for 4 hours. After fixation, the cells were incubated with the affinity purified IgY antibody followed by a FITC-conjugated secondary antibody and analyzed by indirect immunofluorescence.

Acknowledgments

I wish to thank G. Camenisch, D. Chilov, M. Tini, R.H. Wenger, and P. Spielmann for their help in generating and testing chicken antibodies. This project was supported by the Swiss National Science Foundation (31-56743.99).

References

1. Warr, G.W., Magor, K.E., and Higgins, D.A. IgY: clues to the origins of modern antibodies. Immunol Today 1995;16:392.
2. Shimizu, M., Nagashima, H., Sano, K. Hashimoto, K., Ozeki, M., Tsuda, K., and Hatta, H. Molecular stability of chicken and rabbit immunoglobulin G. Biosci Biotechnol Biochem 1992;56:270.
3. Chilov, D., Carnenisch, G., Kvietikova, I., Ziegler, U., Gassmann, M., and Wenger, R.H. Induction and nuclear translocation of hypoxia-inducible factor-1 (HIF-1): heterodimerization with ARNT is not necessary for nuclear accumulation of HIF-1alpha, J Cell Sci 1999;112:1203.
4. Fassina, G., Verdoliva, A., Palambo, G., Ruvo, M. and Cassani, G. Immunoglobulin specificity of TG19318: a novel synthetic ligand for antibody affinity purification. J Mol Recognition 1998;11:128.
5. Murata, T., Saito, S., Shiozaki, M., Lu, R.Z., Eto, Y., Funaba, M., Takahashi, M., and Torii, K. Anti-activin A antibody (IgY) specifically neutralizes various activin A activities. Proc Soc Exp Biol Med 1996;211:100.
6. Gassmann, M., Thömmes, P., Weiser, T., and Hübschr, U. Efficient production of chicken egg yolk antibodies against a conserved mammalian protein. FASEB J 1990;4:2528.
7. Lemamy, G.J., Roger, P., Mani, J.C., Robert, M., Rochefort, H., and Broullet, J.P. High-affinity antibodies from hen's-egg yolks against human mannose-6-phosphate/insulin-like growth-factor-II receptor (M6P/IGFII-R): characterization and potential use in clinical cancer studies. Int J Cancer 1999;80:896.
8. Hensel, T., Amberger, V.R., and Schwab, M.E. A metalloprotease activity from C6 glioma cells inactivates the myelin-associated neurite growth inhibitors and can be neutralized by antibodies. Br J Cancer 1998;78:1564.
9. Almeida, C.M., Kanashiro, M.M., Rangel, Filho, F.B., Mata, M.F., Kipnis, T.L., and da Silva, W.D. Development of snake antivenom antibodies in chickens and their purification from yolk. Vet Rec 1998;143:579.
10. Hatta, H., Tsuda, K., Akachi, S., Kim, M., and Yamamoto, T. Productivity and some properties of egg yolk antibody (IgY) against human rotavirus compared with rabbit IgG. Biosci Biotechnol Biochem 1993;57:450.
11. Wenger, R.H., and Gassmann, M. HIF-1 and the molecular response to hypoxia in mammals. In Environmental Stress and Gene Regulation, Storey, K.B., ed. Oxford: Scientific Publishers Ltd., 1999, chap. 2.
12. Gassmann, M., Kvietikova, L., Rolfs, A., and Wenger, R.H. Oxygen- and dioxin-regulated gene expression in mouse hepatoma cells. Kidney Int 1997;51:567.
13. Gradin, K., McGuire, J., Wenger, R.H., Kvietikova, J., Whitelaw, M.L., Toftgard, R., Tora, L., Gassmann, M., and Poellinger, L. Functional interference between hypoxia and dioxin signal transduction pathways: competition for recruitment of the Arnt transcription factor. Mol Cell Biol 1996;16:5221.

14. Iyer, N.V., Kotch, I.E., Agani, F., Leung, S.W., Laughner, E., Wenger, R.H., Gassmann, M., Gearhart, J.D., Lawler, A.M., Yu, A.Y., and Semenza, G.I. Cellular and developmental control of O_2 homeostasis by hypoxia-inducible factor 1 alpha. Genes Dev 1998;12:149.
15. Carmeliet, P., Dor, Y., Herbert, J.M., Fukumura, D., Brusselmans, K., Dewerchin, M., Neeman, M., Bono, F., Abramovitch, R., Maxwell, P., Koch, C.J., Ratcliffe, P., Moons, L., Jain, R.K., Collen, D., and Keshet, E. Role of HIF-1 alpha in hypoxia-mediated apoptosis, cell proliferation and tumour angiogenesis. Nature 1998;394:485.
16. Ryan, H.E., Lo, J., and Johnson, R.S. HIF-1 alpha is required for solid tumor formation and embryonic vascularization, EMBO J 1998;17:3005.
17. Camenisch, G., Tini, M., Chilov, D., Kvietikova, L., Srinivas, V., Caro, J., and Spielmann, P. General applicability of chicken egg yolk antibodies: the performance of IgY immunoglobulins raised against the hypoxia-inducible factor 1alpha. FASEB J 1999;13:81.
18. Wang, G.L., Jiang, B.H., Rue, E.A., and Semenza, G.L. Hypoxia-inducible factor 1 is a basic-helix-loop-helix-PAS heterodimer regulated by cellular O_2 tension. Proc Natl Acad Sci USA 1995;92:5510.
19. Schwarzkopf, C., and Thiele, B. Chicken IgY: efficacy of alternative adjuvants compared to FCA. In Animal Alternatives, Welfare and Ethics, van Zutphen, L.F.M., Balls, M., eds. Amsterdam: Elsevier Science, 1997, p. 983.
20. Polson, A. Isolation of IgY from the yolks of eggs by a chloroform polyethylene glycol procedure. Immunol Invest 1990;19:253.
21. Fischer, M., Hlinak, A., Montag, T., Claros, M., Schade, R., and Ebner, D. Comparison of standard methods for the preparation of egg yolk antibodies. Tierarztl Prax 1996;24:411.
22. Hansen, P., Scoble, J.A. Hanson, R., and Hoogenraad, N.J. Isolation and purification of immunoglobulins from chicken eggs using thiophilic interaction chromatography. J Immunol Methods 1998;215:1.
23. Kvietikova, I., Wenger, R.H., Marti, H.H., and Gassmann, M. The transcription factors ATF-1 and CREB-1 bind constitutively to the hypoxia-inducible factor-1 (HIF-1) DNA recognition site. Nucleic Acids Res 1995;23:4542.

Section 2

Cholesterol and Health: Role of Eggs

8

Eggs, Plasma Cholesterol, and Heart Disease Risk

Donald J. McNamara

One of the problems is that strong recommendations have often been made on very weak data. It may have been the best guess at the moment. But often the recommendations are repeated so many times that people forget they were rough guesses in the first place and come to think they are hard facts.

—Walter Willett, M.D.
Harvard School of Public Health
(Associated Press 2000)

INTRODUCTION

The public's perception of the role of eggs in the diet has changed dramatically over the last 50 years, going from the view of their being an important contributor of high-quality protein and a variety of vitamins and minerals to the diet to that of their being a major factor in high blood cholesterol levels and increased risk of coronary heart disease (CHD). During the last decade there has been a gradual shift away from the cholesterol-laden "poison pellet" view of eggs toward a more positive one based on the accumulation of extensive evidence indicating that eggs are not a contributor to CHD risk in the population. Indeed, during the same time period that research has made it clear that dietary cholesterol is not the cause of high blood cholesterol, studies have shown that eggs make valuable contributions to the nutritional balance and variety of the diet and that a number of egg components are essential for health maintenance.

The simplicity of the perceived relationship between cholesterol in food and cholesterol in blood had major effects on the dietary patterns of the population and delayed for many years initiation of effective population-based dietary interventions aimed at lowering high blood cholesterol levels and the associated risk of CHD. Even today, the recommendation to restrict weekly egg consumption is widely disseminated to populations around the world in an overly simplistic prescription to lower plasma cholesterol levels. Unfortunately, in too many cases this recommendation is given to low-income populations who subsequently, and needlessly, avoid an affordable source of high-quality protein and nutrients in their diets.

This chapter analyzes the evidence from animal studies; epidemiological surveys, both case-control and prospective; and clinical trials for a relationship between dietary cholesterol (i.e., egg consumption) and CHD risk as assessed by an increase in plasma cholesterol levels, development of atherosclerosis, or fatal and nonfatal CHD.

Lines of Evidence

Various lines of evidence are needed to evaluate the validity and significance of the hypothesized relationship between eggs, dietary cholesterol, and CHD risk. The evidence for a relationship between dietary factors and disease risk is based on the results from animal studies, epidemiological surveys, clinical studies, and the "gold standard" of randomized controlled clinical trials. These lines of evidence have strengths as well as considerable limitations. They can be used either to refute or support a dietary recommendation; however, it is only through consistency of the findings and of the interpretations that they can be used to support or reject specific public health recommendations and policies.

Animal Studies

From the early cholesterol-feeding studies in rabbits showing increased atherosclerosis[1] to the cholesterol-feeding studies in nonhuman primates,[2] one observation is consistent: there is an immense species-to-species variability in the plasma cholesterol response to dietary cholesterol. Some animals are extremely hypersensitive to the hypercholesterolemic effects of dietary cholesterol, while others require feeding pharmacological doses of cholesterol to achieve even small increases in plasma cholesterol concentrations. Conceptually there is clearly a difference between animal feeding studies designed to study the processes of atherogenesis, which often involve diets with extreme levels of both saturated fatty acids and cholesterol, and nutritional studies that are specifically designed to test the effects of physiological intakes of dietary components on plasma lipid and lipoprotein levels and their regulation. Too often the animal studies of atherogenesis have been the basis for conclusions dealing with human nutrition, and the finding that feeding the human equivalents of 2 to 3 g of cholesterol per day to animals results in atherosclerosis has been argued as justification for dietary cholesterol restrictions. However, since humans do not consume such massive doses of cholesterol, it is unclear what biological relevance these studies have to human health. The question of whether there is a threshold for the effects of dietary cholesterol on plasma cholesterol in humans has not been answered nor has the fact that such massive intakes overwhelm the intricate regulatory mechanisms maintaining plasma cholesterol levels within a narrow range[3] been fully considered.

Another complication in the interpretation of animal feeding studies is that most animal species have high-density lipoprotein (HDL) cholesterol as the major plasma lipoprotein whereas humans have low-density lipoprotein (LDL) as the primary transport particle for plasma cholesterol. The metabolisms of these two lipoprotein particles are distinct, and the effects of dietary factors on their plasma concentrations specific to the particles.[4] The finding that a diet high in saturated fat and cholesterol increases total cholesterol levels in an animal model may have little relationship to humans in that the observed increase is in both the LDL- and HDL-cholesterol fractions and, in many cases, the major effect is on HDL-cholesterol levels.

Whether there is any relationship between the observed dietary cholesterol–induced changes in the plasma lipoprotein profile of an HDL animal relative to the risk of hypercholesterolemia and CHD in humans has never been satisfactorily resolved. Neither has the question of whether dietary cholesterol–sensitive or –insensitive nonhuman primates[5] better reflect the human condition. Unfortunately, it is relatively easy to argue either side of the dietary cholesterol– blood cholesterol–CHD issue using data from animal feeding studies.[6,7] One fact is clear: it is virtually impossible to interpret and extrapolate the findings from cholesterol-feeding studies in various animal models to estimate the role of dietary cholesterol in human hypercholesterolemia and development of atherosclerosis.

Epidemiological Data

Many epidemiological surveys have reported a positive correlation between dietary cholesterol and either plasma cholesterol levels or CHD incidence. In contrast, other studies have reported no significant relationship between dietary cholesterol and CHD when multiple regression analyses have included saturated fatty acid calories. The reason for this discrepancy is that there is significant colinearity between the percentage of calories from saturated fatty acid and dietary cholesterol intakes, which compromises the use of simple correlation analyses to determine a significant diet-disease relationship.[8] Data from numerous epidemiological surveys have indicated that saturated fat calories are significantly related to CHD incidence[9–11] and the colinearity of saturated fatty acids and cholesterol must be taken into account in any analysis of epidemiological survey data.

Cross-Sectional Studies

Cross-cultural and within-population studies of the relationship between cholesterol in food and CHD incidence are complicated by a number of factors. Many dietary factors are associated with one another, as well as with overall dietary patterns related to the disease under investigation. For example, diets very high in animal products are usually high in saturated fatty acids and cholesterol and are conversely associated with low intake of fruits and vegetables. As noted above, the colinearity of saturated fatty acids and cholesterol in the diet requires that investigations of the relationships between dietary lipids and CHD utilize multiple regression analyses of the data in order to detect significant relationships.[12]

Kromhout et al.[11] recently reported data from the Seven Countries Study concluding that dietary saturated and *trans*fatty acids and dietary cholesterol were important determinants of differences in population rates of CHD. As shown in Table 8.1, in simple regression analyses, both dietary saturated fatty acids (percentage of calories) and cholesterol intakes (mg/1,000 kcal) are significantly related to CHD rates. However, there is a significant intercorrelation between saturated fatty acids and cholesterol in the diet and when the data are analyzed using multiple regression analysis, dietary cholesterol is no longer significantly related to cross-cultural rates of CHD (Table 8.1). Multivariate analyses indicated that population differences in CHD mortality rates were highly related to differences in intakes of saturated fatty acids. Once the data were adjusted for saturated fatty acid intakes, dietary cholesterol was no longer significantly related to CHD. One source of dietary cholesterol that is not associated with a high intake of saturated fatty acids is the egg, which in the United States accounts for approximately one-third of the cholesterol in the diet.[13]

Data from the Multiple Risk Factor Intervention Trial (MRFIT) indicated that neither dietary cholesterol nor egg consumption was related to baseline plasma cholesterol levels. Study participants were and were not on a special diet (Fig. 8.1). A recently reported analysis of data from the National Health and Nutrition Examination Surveys (NHANES) III by Song and Kerver[14] indicated that egg consumption was unrelated to plasma cholesterol levels in men and women (Fig. 8.2). Both of these studies indicate that egg consumption patterns are unrelated to plasma cholesterol levels.

International data for per capita egg consumption and CHD mortality rates indicate a negative relationship, with the countries with the highest per capita consumption (Japan, Mexico, France, and Spain) having the lowest rates of CHD mortality.[8] Per capita egg consumption in Japan is 338 eggs per person per year, which is almost an egg a day in a population exhibiting very low rates of CHD.

Case-Control Studies

There have been a number of reports from case-control studies investigating the relationship between dietary cholesterol intake and plasma cholesterol levels and CHD incidence. In a recent review of 13 case-control studies, Ravnskov[15] reported no significant differences in cholesterol intakes between CHD cases and controls.[8]

Prospective Studies

The Framingham Heart Study has provided extensive data on risk factors for CHD, with over 50 years of studies related to clinical and lifestyle factors with CHD incidence. Data from the Framingham Heart Study has consistently indicated that dietary cholesterol is not related to either plasma LDL-cholesterol levels or CHD incidence. In 1982 Dawber et al.[16] reported that there was no significant relationship between egg consumption in

Table 8.1. Dietary lipids and CHD rates in the Seven Countries Study

	Simple regression		Multiple regression	
Dietary lipid	*r*	*P*	*r*	*P*
Saturated fatty acids (% cal)	0.88	0.0001	0.88	0.0002
Cholesterol (mg/1,000 kcal)	0.55	0.0291		0.985

Source. Reference 11.

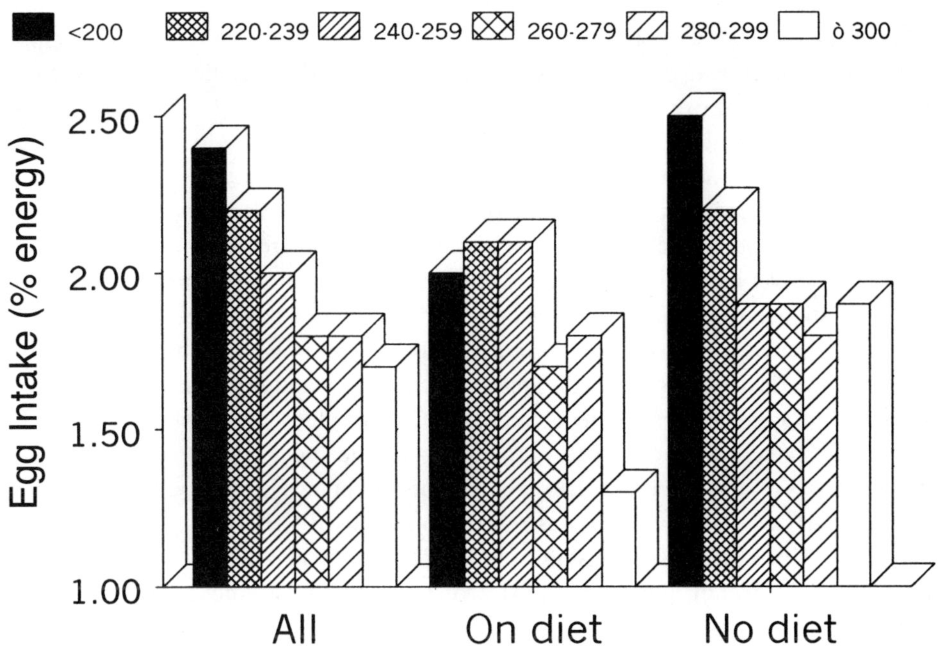

Figure 8.1. Egg consumption and plasma cholesterol levels in MRFIT participants. Adjusted mean percentage of calories from eggs by serum cholesterol concentrations (mg/dl) and special diet status at baseline for 12,553 men in the Multiple Risk Factor Intervention Trial.[25]

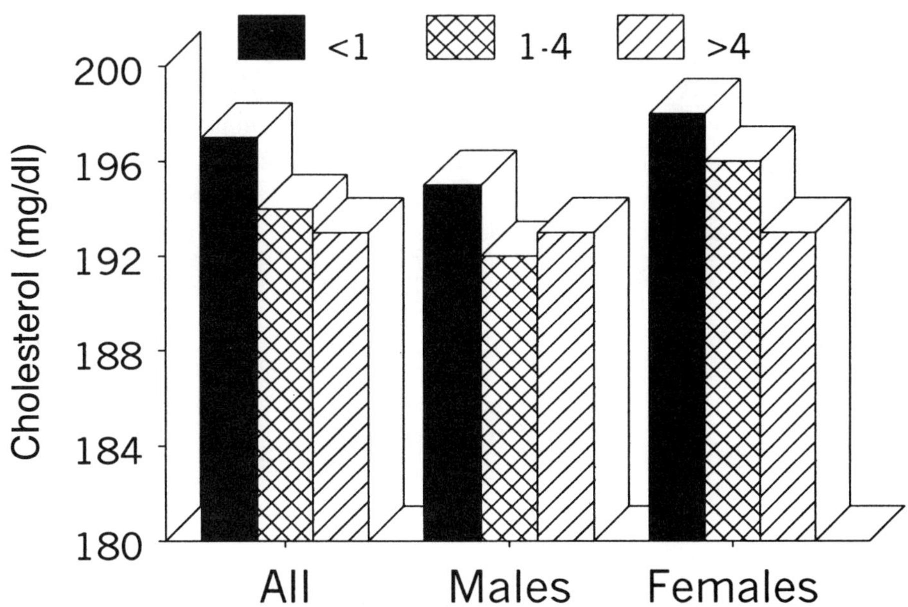

Figure 8.2. Effect of weekly egg consumption on serum cholesterol level (mg/dl). Data from Song and Kerver[14] based on analysis of n = 27,378 NHANES III participants.

the Framingham cohort and either plasma cholesterol levels or CHD incidence.

The largest and most comprehensive study of the relationship between egg consumption and CHD incidence was reported by Hu et al.,[22] who found no relationship between egg consumption and cardiovascular disease in a population of over 177,000 nurses and health professionals followed for 8 to 14 years. There was no difference in CHD relative risk between those who consumed less than one egg a week and those who ate more than one egg a day. The investigators followed 80,082 women for 14 years and 37,851 men for 8 years and looked at the incidence of nonfatal myocardial infarction, fatal coronary heart disease, and stroke incidence as related to daily egg consumption determined by food frequency questionnaires. Weekly egg consumption was unrelated to the relative risk of coronary heart disease in both men and women (Table 8.2). Similar data were obtained for stroke relative risk. Interestingly, the investigators also found no significant increase in relative risk of coronary disease in a small subset of the study group who consumed two or more eggs a day relative to those who never consumed eggs (multivariate relative risk for women was 0.76 and for men 1.1). The authors did note a suggestion that for diabetic subjects higher egg consumption was related to increased CHD risk. The authors concluded that "These findings suggest that consumption of up to 1 egg per day is unlikely to have substantial overall impact on the risk of CHD or stroke among healthy men and women."

This is only one of a long list of recent reports showing that egg consumption and dietary cholesterol intakes are unrelated to either hypercholesterolemia or coronary heart disease incidence. These Harvard investigators also reported that dietary cholesterol was not related to coronary heart disease relative risk in both the Nurses' Health Study (80,082 females)[10] and the Health Professionals Follow-up Study (43,757 males).[9] Similar findings of a nonsignificant relationship between dietary cholesterol and coronary heart disease risk have been reported from the Lipid Research Clinics Follow-up Study (4,546 males and females),[23] the Framingham Heart Study (1,423 females),[17] and the Alpha-Tocopheral, Beta-Carotene Cancer Prevention Study (21,930 males).[24] Over the years a number of investigators have reported a null relationship between egg consumption and plasma lipid

Table 8.2. Egg consumption and CHD risk

	CHD relative risk (95% CI)	
Egg intake/week	Men (n = 37,851)	Women (n = 80,082)
<1	1.0	1.0
1	1.06 (0.88–1.27)	0.82 (0.67–1.00)
2–4	1.12 (0.95–1.33)	0.99 (0.82–1.18)
5–6	0.90 (0.63–1.27)	0.95 (0.70–1.29)
≥7	1.08 (0.79–1.48)	0.82 (0.60–1.13)
P for trends	0.75	0.95

Source. Data for relative risk and 95 percent confidence interval (CI) from Hu et al. Reference 22.

levels as well as between egg intake and coronary heart disease incidence.[25–27] The report by Hu et al.[22] represents the largest epidemiological study to directly relate egg consumption and coronary heart disease risk, and its findings are consistent with the existing literature. No epidemiological studies published in the 1990s have found a significant relationship between dietary cholesterol, or egg consumption, and CHD incidence.[8,28]

Independent Effect

Shekelle and Stamler reported that in the Western Electric Study those individuals in the uppermost quintile of cholesterol intakes had significantly increased relative risk for CHD, even after adjustment for differences in plasma cholesterol concentrations.[29] The level of cholesterol intake in the fifth quintile averaged 1,079 mg/day; the fourth quintile, with an average cholesterol intake of 827 mg/day, was not significantly different from the bottom quintile. In another report, Stamler and Shekelle used data from five epidemiological surveys as further evidence that dietary cholesterol increased CHD risk independent of effects on plasma cholesterol levels;[30] however, in these analyses the CHD relative risks were not adjusted for intake of saturated fatty acids or for plasma cholesterol levels. The data suggest that the overall dietary patterns of study subjects in the top quintile of cholesterol intakes were substantially more atherogenic than just having a high cholesterol intake. This extreme cholesterol intake indicates a very high intake of animal products and, correspondingly, a very low intake of grains, fruits, and vegetables. It can be argued that under these conditions dietary cholesterol simply serves as a surrogate marker for low intakes of grains, vegetables, and fruits in this subset, which would be related to decreased intakes of fiber, antioxidants, and the B vitamins folate, B_6 and B_{12}. Reduced intakes of these nutrients would also increase CHD risk, and the question not addressed in the studies of Stamler and Shekelle[30] is whether the higher CHD incidence in those with the highest cholesterol intakes was due to what was excessive in the diet or, perhaps, what was inadequate in the diet. With today's understanding of the role of antioxidants and B vitamins in CHD risk, it is clear that increased risk occurs not only from nutrient excesses but also from nutrient deficiencies. The potential importance of such confounding dietary variables, which could contribute to the higher CHD incidence in this quintile, was not evaluated by Stamler and colleagues and raises questions regarding the validity of the "independent effect" hypothesis.

Clinical Studies

Cholesterol-feeding studies in humans have been carried out for over 50 years. There are 167 cholesterol-feeding studies in over 3,500 subjects in the scientific literature. In the 1990s a number of reviews have analyzed these studies and reported that the average response to a dietary cholesterol challenge is between 0.022 and 0.025 mg/dl per mg/day cholesterol.[31–35] These analyses have also shown that the dietary cholesterol–mediated increase in plasma total cholesterol results from an increase in both the atherogenic plasma LDL-cholesterol and the antiatherogenic HDL-cholesterol concentrations.[8,35] On average, a 100 mg/day increase in dietary cholesterol would increase plasma total cholesterol by 2.3 mg/dl, plasma LDL-cholesterol by 1.9 mg/dl, and plasma HDL-cholesterol by 0.4 mg/dl. Most cholesterol-feeding studies have reported that dietary cholesterol has little effect on the ratio of plasma LDL- to HDL-cholesterol. The lack of effect of dietary cholesterol on the LDL:HDL ratio is consistent with the epidemiological observations of a null relationship between dietary cholesterol and CHD incidence.

Analysis of the cholesterol-feeding studies in the literature indicates that the plasma cholesterol response to dietary cholesterol is independent of the type or amount of fat in the diet. In contrast, certain physiological and genetic characteristics are associated with an increased sensitivity to dietary cholesterol. Studies indicate that hypercholesterolemic individuals have a smaller plasma cholesterol response to dietary cholesterol than subjects with combined hyperlipidemia. Studies also indicate that patients with certain genetic variants of apolipoprotein E are hyperresponders to dietary cholesterol. The best estimate is that between 15 and 20 percent of the population exhibit a hyperresponse to dietary cholesterol while 80 to 85 percent are hyporesponders to cholesterol intake. Analysis of available data indicates that the plasma cholesterol response to a 100 mg/day change in dietary cholesterol is 1.4 mg/dl in hyporesponders compared with a 3.9 mg/dl change in hyperresponders.[31]

Randomized Control Clinical Trials

There has never been, and probably never will be, a clinical trial to answer the dietary cholesterol–CHD question. The "gold standard" for determining a relationship between a nutrient and a disease will never be applied to the dietary cholesterol–CHD issue and as such there will probably continue to be considerable debate on this topic.

Conclusion

There is only a scattering of weak epidemiological evidence suggesting that dietary cholesterol has a relationship with CHD incidence, and virtually every study reported during the last decade has supported the null hypothesis. The studies that do suggest a positive correlation have usually based this relationship on simple regression analyses of the data and have failed to correct for the colinearity of saturated fat calories and cholesterol intakes. The overwhelming majority of case-control and prospective studies indicate that dietary cholesterol is not a factor in CHD incidence, and the suggestion that dietary cholesterol might be an independent risk factor for CHD is not supported by the available evidence.

There have been a number of recent reviews of the epidemiological and clinical evidence relating dietary cholesterol to plasma cholesterol levels and CHD incidence.[3,8,12,15,28,32,33,36–38] These reviews have consistently arrived at the conclusion that dietary cholesterol is not a factor in CHD incidence. The current state of confusion on the issue is based on conflict between the results of epidemiological surveys indicating no dietary cholesterol–CHD relationship and the clinical feeding trials that find a small increase in plasma cholesterol with cholesterol feeding. The problem is that not all increases in plasma total cholesterol are related to an increase in CHD risk, especially when the intervention, in this case dietary cholesterol, does not alter the LDL:HDL ratio. The data are clear that dietary cholesterol affects both LDL- and HDL-cholesterol levels and that in hyporesponders there is no effect on the ratio of these two markers of CHD risk.

The extent of the evidence that egg consumption was, in fact, not related to CHD risk was sufficient to warrant a change in the American Heart Association (AHA) 30-year-old dietary recommendation that healthy Americans consume no more than three to four whole eggs a week to allow intake of up to seven eggs a week.[39] The AHA Dietary Guidelines 2000 puts an enhanced emphasis on dietary patterns rather than on limits of specific nutrients and not only advises on the dietary factors to be limited but also promotes foods that provide high nutrient density and an associated lower risk of CHD.

Dedication

The author dedicates this review to the memory of E.H. "Pete" Ahrens, Jr., M.D.—physician, scientist, teacher, and mentor. His research helped define the effects of dietary lipids on plasma cholesterol levels, and in the process he trained a generation of clinical investigators. His constant demand for science-based evidence continues to be a model of questioning the conventional wisdom.

References

1. Anitschkow, N., and Chalatow, S. Ueber Experimentelle Cholesterinsteatose und ihre Bedeutung fur die Entstehung einiger pathologischer Prozesse. Zentralbl Allg Pathol Anat 1913;24:1.
2. Rudel, L.L. Genetic factors influence the atherogenic response of lipoproteins to dietary fat and cholesterol in nonhuman primates. J Am Coll Nutr 1997;16:306.
3. McNamara, D.J. Dietary cholesterol: effects on lipid metabolism. Curr Opin Lipidol 1990;1:18.
4. Fernandez, M.L., Wilson, T.A., Conde, K., Vergara-Jimenez, M., and Nicolosi, R.J. Hamsters and guinea pigs differ in their plasma lipoprotein cholesterol distribution when fed diets varying in animal protein, soluble fiber, or cholesterol content. J Nutr 1999;129:1323.
5. Clarkson, T.B., Bond, M.G., Bullock, B.C., McLaughlin, K.J., and Sawyer, J.K. A study of atherosclerosis regression in *Macaca mullata*. V. Changes in abdominal aorta and carotid and coronary arteries from animals with atherosclerosis induced for 38 months and then regressed for 24 or 48 months at plasma cholesterol concentrations of 300 or 200 mg/dl. Exp Mol Pathol 1984;41:96.
6. McNamara, D.J. Dietary cholesterol, serum cholesterol, and risks of cardiovascular and noncardiovascular diseases—reply, Am J Clin Nutr 1998;67:491.
7. Stamler, J., Greenland, P., Van Horn, L., and Grundy, S.M. Dietary cholesterol, serum cholesterol, and risks of cardiovascular and noncardiovascular diseases. Am J Clin Nutr 1998;67:488.
8 McNamara, D.J. Dietary cholesterol and atherosclerosis. Biochim Biophys Acta 2000;1529:310.
9. Ascherio, A., Rimm, E.B., Giovannucci, E.L., Spiegelman, D., Stampfer, M., and Willett, W.C. Dietary fat and risk of coronary heart disease in men: cohort follow up study in the United States. BMJ 1996;313:84.
10. Hu, F.B., Stampfer, M.J., Manson, J.E., Rimm, E., Colditz, G.A., Rosner, B.A., Hennekens,

C.H., and Willett, W.C. Dietary fat intake and the risk of coronary heart disease in women. N Engl J Med 1997;337:1491.

11. Kromhout, D., Menotti, A., Bloemberg, B., Aravanis, C., Blackburn, H., Buzina, R., Dontas, A.S., Fidanza, F., Giampaoli, S., Jansen, A., et al. Dietary saturated and trans fatty acids and cholesterol and 25-year mortality from coronary heart disease: the Seven Countries Study. Prev Med 1995;24:308.
12. Hegsted, D.M., and Ausman, L.M. Diet, alcohol and coronary heart disease in men. J Nutr 1988;118:1184.
13. Federation of American Societies for Experimental Biology. Report on Nutrition Monitoring in the United States. Vol. 1. Washington, DC: U.S. Government Printing Office, 1995.
14. Song, W.O., and Kerver, J.M. Nutritional contribution of eggs to American diets. J Am Coll Nutr 2000;19:556S.
15. Ravnskov, U. Quotation bias in reviews of the diet-heart idea. J Clin Epidemiol 1995;48:713.
16. Dawber, T.R., Nickerson, R.J., Brand, F.N., and Pool, J. Eggs, serum cholesterol, and coronary heart disease. Am J Clin Nutr 1982;36:617.
17. Millen, B.E., Franz, M.M., Quatromoni, P.A., Gagnon, D.R., Sonnenberg, L.M., Ordovas, J.M., Wilson, P.W.F., Schaefer, E.J., and Cupples, L.A. Diet and plasma lipids in women. 1. Macronutrients and plasma total and low-density lipoprotein cholesterol in women: the Framingham nutrition studies. J Clin Epidemiol 1996;49:657.
18. Posner, B.M. On the importance of dietary fat. Conclusions from the Framingham Study. Acta Cardiol 1993;48:452.
19. Posner, B.M., Cobb, J.L., Belanger, A.J., Cupples, L.A., D'Agostino, R.B., and Stokes, J.D. Dietary lipid predictors of coronary heart disease in men. The Framingham Study. Arch Intern Med 1991;151:1181.
20. Posner, B.M., Cupples, L.A., Franz, M.M., and Gagnon, D.R. Diet and heart disease risk factors in adult American men and women: the Framingham offspring-spouse nutrition studies. Int J Epidemiol 1993;22:1014.
21. Posner, B.M., Cupples, L.A., Miller, D.R., Cobb, J.L., Lutz, K.J., and D'Agostino, R.B. Diet, menopause, and serum cholesterol levels in women: the Framingham Study. Am Heart J 1993;125:483.
22. Hu, F.B., Stampfer, M.J., Rimm, E.B., Manson, J.E., Ascherio, A., Colditz, G.A., Rosner, B.A., Spiegelman, D., Speizer, F.E., Sacks, F.R., Hennekens, C.H., and Willett, W.C. A prospective study of egg consumption and risk of cardiovascular disease in men and women. JAMA 1999;281:1387.
23. Esrey, K.L., Joseph, L., and Grover, S.A. Relationship between dietary intake and coronary heart disease mortality: lipid research clinics prevalence follow-up study. J Clin Epidemiol 1996;49:211.
24. Pietinen, P., Ascherio, A., Korhonen, P., Hartman, A.M., Willett, W.C., Albanes, D., and Virtamo, J. Intake of fatty acids and risk of coronary heart disease in a cohort of Finnish men—the alpha-tocopherol, beta-carotene cancer prevention study. Am J Epidemiol 1997;145:876.
25. Tillotson, J.L., Bartsch, G.E., Gorder, D., Grandits, G.A., and Stamler, J. Food group and nutrient intakes at baseline in the Multiple Risk Factor Intervention Trial. Am J Clin Nutr 1997;65(Suppl.):228S.
26. Gramenzi, A., Gentile, A., Fasoli, M., Negri, E., Parazzini, F., and La Vecchia, C. Association between certain foods and risk of acute myocardial infarction in women. BMJ 1990;300:771.
27. Fraser, G.E. Diet and coronary heart disease: beyond dietary fats and low-density-lipoprotein cholesterol. Am J Clin Nutr 1994;59:1117S.

28. McNamara, D.J. Eggs, dietary cholesterol and heart disease risk: an international perspective. In Egg Nutrition and Biotechnology, Sim, J.S., Nakai, S., and Guenter, W., eds. New York: CABI Publishing, 1999, p. 55.
29. Shekelle, R.B., and Stamler, J. Dietary cholesterol and ischaemic heart disease. Lancet 1989;I:1177.
30. Stamler, J., and Shekelle, R. Dietary cholesterol and human coronary heart disease. The epidemiological evidence. Arch Pathol Lab Med 1988;112:1032.
31. McNamara, D.J. The impact of egg limitations on coronary heart disease risk: Do the numbers add up? J Am Coll Nutr 2000;19:540S.
32. McNamara, D. Cholesterol intake and plasma cholesterol: an update. J Am Coll Nutr 1997;16:530.
33. McNamara, D.J. Relationship between blood and dietary cholesterol. Adv Meat Res 1990;6:63.
34. Howell, W.H., McNamara, D.J., Tosca, M.A., Smith, B.T., and Gaines, J.A. Plasma lipid and lipoprotein responses to dietary fat and cholesterol: a meta-analysis. Am J Clin Nutr 1997;65:1747.
35. Clarke, R., Frost, C., Collins, R., Appleby, P., and Peto, R. Dietary lipids and blood cholesterol: quantitative meta-analysis of metabolic ward studies. BMJ 1997;314:112.
36. McNamara, D.J. Dietary cholesterol and the optimal diet for reducing risk of atherosclerosis. Can J Cardiol 1995;11(Suppl. G):123G.
37. Kritchevsky, S.B., and Kritchevsky, D. Egg consumption and coronary heart disease: an epidemiologic overview. J Am Coll Nutr 2000;19:549S.
38. Hegsted, D.M., Ausman, L.M., Johnson, J.A., and Dallal, G.E. Dietary fat and serum lipids: an evaluation of the experimental data. Am J Clin Nutr 1993;57:875.
39. Krauss, R.M., Eckel, R.H., Howard, B.V., Appel, L.J., Daniels, S.R., Deckelbaum, R.J., Erdman, J.W., Jr., Kris-Etherton, P., Goldberg, I.J., Kotchen, T.A., Lichtenstein, A.H., Mitch, W.E., Mullis, R., Robinson, K., Wylie-Rosett, J., St. Jeor, S., Suttie, J., Tribble, D.L., and Bazzarre, T.L. AHA Dietary Guidelines. Revision 2000: A statement for healthcare professionals from the Nutrition Committee of the American Heart Association. Circulation 2000;102:2296.

9

Eggs and Health: Myths and Misconceptions

Simin Bolourchi Vaghefi

Nutritional Benefits of Eggs

Eggs are one of the highest–nutrient-dense foods with the most economic value. A large egg contains 6 g of protein, of which approximately 3 g are in the yolk and 3 g in white. An egg also contains 5 g of fat, 28 mg of calcium, 317 mg of vitamin A, 1 mg of iron, 0.55 mg of zinc, and B vitamins such as thiamin, riboflavin, niacin, B_6, folic acid, vitamin B_{12}, and vitamins D and E.

Eggs are very nutrient dense. Nutrient density is the ratio of nutrients to calories. An egg contains varying amounts of 13 vitamins, many minerals, and about 80 calories per egg. Eggs are an ideal food to be included in the diet of those who wish to limit their energy intake but receive the important nutrients that their body requires. The size of the egg determines the number of calories. A medium egg provides 66 calories, while a jumbo egg has 94 calories. Large and extra large eggs have 75 and 84 calories respectively.

It is obvious that no one food (other than mother's milk) provides every nutrient needed by human infants. Eggs contain a wide variety of essential nutrients including essential amino acids in addition of the above mentioned vitamins and minerals in a ratio very close to the requirement of humans. Large eggs, which cost about 10 cents each, are certainly one of the most inexpensive foods that provides large numbers and amounts of nutrients. Thus it is a very efficient food to include in the diets of two groups of people:

1. Those people who wish to control their weight or lose the extra weight they carry can use eggs as a source of many nutrients and reduce their intake of high-fat, high-calorie foods such as meat, whole milk, and high-fat dairy products like cheese and ice cream. To limit calories, eggs can be substituted for meat in diets with low fat content and high fiber, high concentrated carbohydrates, adequate fruits and vegetables, and skim dairy products. This type of diet is very effective and practical in reducing unwanted body fat, provided physical activity is also included.
2. People of low economic status can use eggs as a source of many nutrients at a very economical price.

Eggs are a versatile food that can be used in combination with other food groups to help provide variety in the diet. Lactoovovegetarians use eggs in place of meat in variety of recipes, by combining it with vegetables in omelets, soups, stews, and rice and other cereals, as an appetizer, a main dish, or a desert.

Egg Protein

Eggs have the highest-quality protein, with the amino acid pattern almost matching the human requirements for essential amino acids. For this reason egg protein is used as the standard for evaluating the quality of protein in other foods. FAO nutrition experts have given egg protein a value of 100 for the presence of all essential amino acids with almost the proportion to the human need in egg white.[1]

Mother's milk provides the exact proportion of essential amino acids required by human infants for growth. Egg protein is next to mother's milk in that respect.

Digestibility of egg protein is 97 percent. This means that 97 percent of the egg's proteins are absorbed by the human intestine in the form of amino acids. The absorbed amino acids are available (1) for new protein synthesis in the body for growth and maintenance of the tissues and (2) to replace the lost proteins. This puts egg protein higher than any other food in terms of digestibility and biological availability.

The biological value of egg protein is 94 percent. That indicates protein quality of high efficiency rate. Biological value is the measure of the rate at which the protein in food supports growth. The biological value of whole egg protein is about 93.7, milk is next with a biological value of 84.5, meats in general have the biological value of about 75, rice and wheat's biological value is 64.[2] Eggs and milk have the highest biological value and provide more amino acids for growth and tissue maintenance than even meat, including beef, chicken, pork, and fish. This gives the egg protein a very high nutritional value.

Evenepoel and colleagues studied the digestibility of raw and cooked egg proteins in ileostomy patients. The patients ingested 25 g of egg protein labeled with ^{13}C and ^{15}N to evaluate the egg protein assimilation by both the ^{13}C breath test technique and the direct analysis of the ileostomy effluents. They established that heat treatment of egg proteins enhances their digestibility. In this study it was demonstrated that cooked egg protein had a digestibility of 90.9 percent +/- 0.8 and the digestibility of raw egg protein was 51.3 +/-9.8 percent.[3] Raw egg consumption is rare. Especially for health reasons eggs should be consumed cooked.

Egg Fat

Eggs contain about 5 to 6 g of fat depending on the size. One-third or about 1.5 g of egg fat are saturated and two-thirds or about 3.5 g are unsaturated. Fatty acids, which are the basic chemical units of fat, are either saturated, monounsaturated, or polyunsaturated. It has been shown that saturated fats increase cholesterol synthesis by the liver cells and result in elevation of blood LDL (low-density lipoprotein) -cholesterol.

Monounsaturated fatty acids and polyunsaturated fatty acids tend to decrease blood cholesterol levels. Polyunsaturated fatty acids are found primarily in fats of plant origin and in fats of fatty fish.

The cholesterol content of eggs is rather high, about 210 mg. Although egg cholesterol content has been reported to be 185, 200, 215, 218 or 300 mg, the generally used figure is an average of about 200 mg/egg. The high cholesterol content of eggs has caused health professionals to caution people, especially those who are susceptible to cardiovascular disease, to reduce the consumption of eggs to no more than four yolks a week. This advice has caused many health conscious individuals to avoid eating eggs completely and leave this nutritious food out of their diet.

Egg White

Egg white protein is mostly albumen, which accounts for 67 percent of egg protein. The egg white contains, in addition to protein, niacin, riboflavin, chlorine, magnesium, potassium, sodium, and sulfur. The albumen forms four alternating layers of thick and thin consistencies. From the yolk outward, they are designated as the inner thick white, the inner thin white, the outer thick white, and the outer thin white. Egg white tends to thin out as an egg ages because its protein changes in character. That's why fresh eggs sit up tall and firm in the pan while older ones tend to spread out.

Albumen is more opalescent than truly white. The cloudy appearance comes from carbon dioxide. As the egg ages, carbon dioxide dissolved in the egg white escapes, so the albumen of older eggs is more transparent than that of fresher eggs.

When egg albumen is beaten vigorously, it foams and increases in volume six to eight times as the protein is denatured. Egg foams are extensively used for making soufflés, meringues, puffy omelets, and angel food and sponge cakes.

Egg Yolk

The yolk or yellow portion makes up about 33 percent of the liquid weight of the egg. It contains all of the fat in the egg and a little less than half of the protein.

The yolk contains a higher proportion of the egg's vitamins than the white. Except for riboflavin and niacin, which are higher in the white than in the yolk. Vitamins A, D, and E, being fat soluble, are contained in the fat of the yolk. Egg yolks are one of the few foods naturally containing vitamin D.

The yolk's content of phosphorus, manganese, iron, iodine, copper, and calcium are higher than the white's, and it contains all of the zinc. The yolk of a large egg contains about 59 calories.

Young hens whose egg production cycles are not yet completely established may produce double-yolk eggs. These types of eggs are also often produced by hens that are old enough to produce extra large eggs. It is thought that genetics is a factor too. Occasionally a hen will produce double-yolk eggs throughout her egg-laying career. It is rare, but not unknown, for a young hen to produce an egg with no yolk at all. In fertilized eggs, the yolk is the site of embryo formation. The nutrient in the yolk and white portion of the egg provides for the growth of the embryo.

The lecithin in the yolk is responsible for the egg's emulsifying properties. The heat of cooking causes some minor nutrient loss in the egg. Riboflavin, thiamin, and folic acid contained in the egg are generally less heat stable than other nutrients. Normal cooking denatures the egg protein, but it is still just as nutritious and contains all of the amino acids that make up the protein. Amino acids are destroyed only when eggs are severely overcooked, such as in the brown lacy edges of an overcooked fried egg. If overcooking is avoided, egg nutrients as well as amino acids of the egg protein are preserved.

Nutrient Composition of Eggs

According to the data from the U.S. Department of Agriculture, nutrition value of one large raw egg is as follows:

Of the 38 g of water in one large egg, 29 g are in the white, and 9 gram in the yolk. The calorie content of whole egg is 75. Seventeen calories are from egg white, and 58 calories from the yolk. Of the 6.25 g egg protein, 3.5 g are in the white, and 2.75 g in the yolk. As was mentioned earlier all of the 5 g of fat are in the yolk. The 0.61 g of carbohydrate are equally divided in yolk and white.

Breakdown of the lipids in the yolk is as follows: Fatty acids as triacylglycerides, 4.3 g; total saturated fat, 1.6 g; total monounsaturated fat, 1.9 g; and 0.7 g of polyunsaturated oil (1.1 g palmetic acid and 1.7 g oleic acid). A large egg also contains 215 mg of cholesterol and 0.6 gram of linoleic acid.[3] Cholesterol content of the egg is recorded differently, according to the source. Figures of 300 mg, 218 mg, 200 mg, and 185 mg appear in the literature.

Egg Vitamins and Minerals

Vitamin analysis of the egg is described as follows: Fat-soluble vitamins A, D, and E are present in the yolk at 317, 25, and 0.7 mg respectively. Water-soluble vitamins of the egg include B_{12}, 0.50 mcg; biotin, 9.98 mcg; folacin, 24 mcg; pyridoxine, 0.07 mg; riboflavin, 0.254 mg, and thiamine, 0.031 mg.

Biotin is a B vitamin that plays an important role in cell metabolism and the utilization of fats, proteins, and carbohydrates. Biotin is present in many foods, including egg yolk, and is synthesized by the intestinal bacteria in the body. One of the raw egg proteins is avidin. This protein can combine with biotin and make it biologically unavailable. However, a human would have to eat 24 raw egg whites a day for biotin to be inhibited by avidin. Heat inactivates the avidin, and most eggs are served cooked

Breakdown of the mineral content of the egg is as follows: calcium, 25 mg; iodine, 0.024 mg; iron, 0.72 mg; magnesium, 5 mg; manganese, 0.013 mg; phosphorus, 89 mg; potassium, 64 mg; sodium, 63 mg; and zinc, 0.55 mg.[4]

Eggs and Nutrition

As one looks at nutrients and their amounts in eggs, it becomes obvious that including eggs in one's diet helps to meet many of the nutrients' requirements. Eggs are a very economic food at about $0.10 each. Three eggs can be substituted for one serving of meat (one egg being equivalent of one ounce of meat) with most of the nutrients and a fraction of the price, about 30 cents. Obviously eggs can provide good nutrition in a very inexpensive way for people living in poverty. Eggs are, for this reason, on the list of special supplemental foods for recipients of the Women, Infants, and Children (WIC) program.

Families with limited income can derive their needed nutrients by including eggs in their diet. Added to the diet of vegetarians, eggs will provide nutrients they might be deficient in, such as iron, vitamin B_{12}, magnesium, and zinc. Added to the diet of pregnant women and young children who may suffer from iron deficiency anemia will provide protein as well as iron, folacin, and B_{12} to overcome that deficiency. It is reported that 15 percent of the children and pregnant women in the world suffer from iron deficiency anemia. Most of these people live in poverty and suffer from deficiency of not only iron but protein and other minerals as well as vitamins.

Unfortunately, eggs have been blamed for their cholesterol content and wrongfully targeted for restriction in the diet of Western industrialized countries. Underdeveloped and developing countries of the world look for scientific, health, nutritional, and medical information from vast research institutions in the West. Therefore, in many of these countries consumption of eggs is restricted to the levels recommended by the American Heart Association or other health and medical organizations.

Following the recommendations to restrict the consumption of eggs means depriving a great number of individuals who may not be at the risk of cardiovascular diseases (CVDs). These restrictions were recommended for people who are at risk of death from CVDs. It is now established that risks for CVDs are many and, as research indicates, consumption of eggs is the least of those risk factors.

After all, a small percentage of the population either inherits the risk factors for CVDs or has a lifestyle conducive to acquiring these risks. In these times when most people in the industrial countries are conscious of their health and monitor it, the blanket recommendation to limit consumption of eggs is not justified—especially when it is becoming clear that the dietary cholesterol of eggs is not responsible for increasing the plasma levels of cholesterol in normal individuals

According to egg industry data, average per capita consumption of eggs in 1945 was 405 eggs per year. The average per capita consumption of eggs has declined to about 235. These averages undoubtedly include people who consume large numbers of eggs each day, people who do not eat eggs at all, and those who consume about one egg a day. However, the reduction in average egg consumption is an indication that the population has taken the egg restriction advice to heart and is following it. As research indicates, individuals vary in their plasma cholesterol response to dietary fat and cholesterol. Genetics, ethnicity, body weight, fat distribution in the body, and physical activity are factors that determine the response of plasma total and LDL-cholesterol to the dietary fat and cholesterol in healthy subjects.

Myths and Misconceptions about Eggs

One of the most important risk factors for coronary heart disease is elevated low-density lipoprotein cholesterol (LDL-C).[5] In many experimental animals dietary cholesterol increases levels of LDL-C and causes atherosclerosis. Dietary cholesterol elevates the level of blood total and LDL-cholesterol in human subjects as shown in controlled metabolic studies.[6,7] Elevation of serum cholesterol in response to increased dietary saturated fat and transfatty acids is significantly higher.[8] Studies have shown that there are wide variations in individual serum cholesterol response to dietary cholesterol. There are studies, however, showing that dietary cholesterol has very little effect on plasma cholesterol levels. Research reports are equally divided on the question of positive or negative plasma cholesterol response to dietary cholesterol.

Reports of studies that indicated a relationship between the dietary cholesterol and CVDs have caused many people fearing the cardiovascular diseases to forgo eggs as a nutritious part of their diets. However, there is a considerable amount of accumulated research data over the last 30 some years showing that dietary cholesterol has a very small effect on plasma levels of cholesterol. Still, these research results have not changed the debate on whether dietary cholesterol is responsible for the increase in the level of plasma cholesterol and risk of cardiovascular diseases. Recent research has provided ample evidence that dietary cholesterol has little relation to the plasma cholesterol levels and the risk of heart disease. The research has elucidated that, after all, eggs are not a bad food. In fact eggs are a very nutritious food.

After reviewing several studies, McNamara in 1997 showed that adding one or two eggs per day to a low-fat diet had no effect on blood cholesterol levels. Data obtained from the reviewed studies showed that young men and women as well as older subjects could add one or two eggs per day to their diet and not increase their blood cholesterol level. In this review the population-wide restriction of eggs to no more that three to four per week is questioned.[9]

It is interesting but disappointing that food venders have resorted to labeling food as cholesterol-free to profit from this phobia that is so common in the population. Eggs have been associated with high cholesterol ever since the cholesterol content was reported to be 300 mg. Later that figure was reduced to 218, 215, and 200 mg depending on the source of the data.

Restricting consumption of eggs because of high cholesterol content has become a part of dietary practices of the American public. As a result many health conscious individuals and families have joined the egg phobia/dietary cholesterol phobia culture, restricting their consumption of eggs and other high cholesterol–containing foods. It would be much more beneficial, health wise, if people would reduce their intake of fast food and other high-fat and saturated fat foods.

In the industrialized countries, especially in the United States, people partake of a great amount of fast foods and convenience foods. Both of these food categories contain very high amounts of fat, especially saturated fat, transfatty acids, and high cholesterol. The average fat content of the diet of Americans is 37 to 38 percent of the daily energy intake. While the recommendation to restrict eggs in the diet is observed by many, other recommendations of the American Heart Association are virtually ignored, such as reducing fat, especially saturated and transfatty acid intake, and increasing fiber in the diet by consuming more cereals, vegetables, and fruits. This is clearly evidenced by the dietary fat intake reported from the NHANES II data.[10]

The recommendation to restrict eggs in the diet contradicts the vast number of the studies published and the abundant data available regarding risk factors for CVDs. Research reports showing that dietary cholesterol and consumption of eggs increase the risk for CVDs are countered by a large body of data available indicating that atherosclerotic diseases are related to many other factors. These factors, which can be a risk for CVDs alone or in combination, are hypertension, obesity, circulating blood lipids, the ratio of low-density lipoprotein cholesterol (LDL-C) to high-density lipoprotein cholesterol (HDL-C), smoking, alcohol consumption, a sedentary lifestyle, stressful living, and genetic factors.[11,12] The one factor that is of extreme importance is the amount of cholesterol that is carried around in the bloodstream by low-density lipoproteins. These specific groups of circulating plasma lipids and their oxidation by reactive oxygen appear to be directly related to the incidences of the disease.[13]

As a result of these findings and concerns about the fact that cardiovascular diseases, together, make up the number one killer disease in the West, health officials blamed dietary cholesterol for heart disease and recommended reducing foods with high cholesterol content. This idea is now being challenged by many new research reports indicating that dietary cholesterol has very little effect on LDL-cholesterol.

Numerous studies with both experimental animals and human subjects have shown that the level of circulating LDL-C is directly related to the amount of saturated fatty acids in the diet. Increased consumption of saturated fat will elevate the level of circulating LDL-C in the blood, while consumption of mono- and polyunsaturated fatty acids in the diet will result in reduction of the LDL-C. When a diet contains equal amount of both types of fatty acids, saturated fats cause the level of LDL-C to increase, rendering polyunsaturated fat unable to lower the levels of LDL-C.[14,15] It can be concluded that saturated fatty acids are the culprit and they should be limited in the diet.

Interestingly one of the Dietary Guidelines for American Adults is to reduce consumption of saturated fatty acids to 10 percent of energy intake, which is being ignored by the population. This may be because it is not easy to change dietary habits, but it is very easy to restrict or eliminate one food item from the diet. If this is the case, in order to reduce the morbidity and mortality from CVDs, and remove CVDs as the number one cause of death in the West, a whole new method must be thought out to educate people and convince them that if they wish to avoid cardiovascular diseases, they need to change their eating habits and lifestyle.

Mattson et al. reported that the level of circulating LDL-C is responsive to dietary cholesterol. In other words LDL-C levels are increased when dietary cholesterol is increased.[16] Other reports indicate that plasma cholesterol is elevated with an increase in dietary cholesterol, especially when the intake of dietary saturated fatty acids are increased.[17] The elevation of plasma cholesterol varies considerably among individuals. The increase in plasma cholesterol levels also varies in distribution among the plasma lipoprotein fractions. That dietary cholesterol only raises the plasma levels of LDL-C can be questioned since other studies have shown that increase in both LDL and HDL lipoprotein cholesterol is possible in response to dietary cholesterol.[18] Body fat distribution as well as gender and age are factors that determine the effect of dietary fatty acids and cholesterol on the increased plasma lipoproteins.[19]

It is not only the level of LDL-C circulating in the blood that increases the risk of atherosclerosis. There are many factors that can influence oxidation of this lipoprotein and cause it to adhere to the inner surface of the arteries, raising the incidence of arteriosclerosis. These factors include, in general, high composition of saturated fatty acids of animal origin in the diet and the variety and amounts and types of the antioxidants and photochemicals that an individual receives from his or her diet that can prevent the oxidation of the LDL-cholesterol. This is one of the reasons that consumption of fruits and vegetables is emphasized.

Many of the antioxidants such as α-tocopherol, vitamin C, and β-carotene are present in eggs. Eggs also add to the variety in a diet since they can be used in combination with a number of food items.

Cholesterol Synthesis and Metabolism

In order to best understand the effect or lack of effect of dietary cholesterol on plasma total cholesterol and LDL-C, a brief description of cholesterol synthesis and metabolism is given below.

Dietary cholesterol that comes only from animal products is absorbed from the intestine along with dietary fat, incorporated into chylomicron and transported to the liver.[20,21] As the level of cholesterol in the liver increases, the rate of cholesteryl ester synthesis is increased. The rate of hepatic cholesterol synthesis from acetyl CoA is partially suppressed.[22] Cholesterol is also synthesized in nearly all of the other extrahepatic tissues, but the rates are different in each tissue. Cholesterol synthesized by these tissues is equal to the amount transported to the liver by high-density lipoprotein (HDL).[23]

Loss of cholesterol from the body is mainly through the bile acids or bile salts excretion in the intestine to aid digestion of fat. These bile acids are then reabsorbed and carried to the liver. Consumption of a diet high in insoluble fiber causes the bile to be adsorbed to the surface of insoluble fiber and excreted in the feces, interrupting the enterohepatic circulation of sterols. This is the only major route for cholesterol excretion. Consumption of a low-fiber diet does not interrupt the cycle and allows the bile salts to be reabsorbed and carried to the liver. A very small amount of cholesterol is also lost through the sloughing of the skin and endothelial tissue.

There is usually a balance of cholesterol as the amount of sterols that exit the body as bile acids are equal to cholesterol synthesized by the liver and extrahepatic tissues as well as that absorbed from the diet. The liver synthesis of cholesterol will change to maintain the balance of cholesterol. For example on days when the dietary cholesterol is high, the rate of hepatic cholesterol synthesis decreases. Thus, it is the change in the rate of synthesis in the liver that maintains the balance and not the extrahepatic synthesis of cholesterol. It has been well established that the liver plays a central role in keeping the balance of cholesterol or sterol in the body by increasing cholesterol synthesis when fecal cholesterol excretion in the form of bile acids increases and by inhibiting synthesis when fecal losses are minimal.

Cholesterol is mostly circulated in the liver in the form of LDL-C. Liver cells LDL-C receptors actively take up the LDL-C for metabolism. Other extrahepatic tissues also contain LDL-C receptors that are not as active as the liver cell receptors. Thus, plasma concentration of LDL-C is greatly affected by the rate at which LDL-C is formed and the rate of uptake by LDL-C receptors.[13] Therefore, genetics plays a role here by determining the rate of activity of LDL-C receptors.

The liver is the organ that receives most of the absorbed cholesterol and part of the absorbed triacylglycerols. It is the liver that regulates metabolism of the lipids and maintains the balance of cholesterol and circulating LDL-C. The lipids entering hepatocytes affect the distribution of fatty acids in cholesterol esters triacylglycerols and phospholipids (components of membrane lipids of the cells). Also they alter the cholesterol pool of the cells. All of these changes affect the changes in LDL receptors' activity and LDL-C production by the liver.[24]

It has been proven that consumption of a diet high in saturated fatty acids (diets high in animal foods contain saturated fatty acids) raises the blood levels of cholesterol. It has also been shown that consumption of large amounts of mono- and polyunsaturated fatty acids reduces the plasma levels of cholesterol. Kris-Etherton et al. showed that a diet high in monounsaturated fatty acids can lower both plasma total and LDL-cholesterol levels but have no effect on plasma HDL-cholesterol or triacylglycerol concentrations. In this investigation 22 subjects participated in a five-period crossover study. Over the five periods they consumed several diets: (1) An average American diet (AAD), containing 50 percent of the calories as carbohydrates (CHOs), 16 percent as protein, 34 percent as fat of which 16 percent was saturated fatty acids (SFAs), 11 percent monounsaturated fatty acids (MUFAs), and 7 percent polyunsaturated fatty acids (PUFAs). (2) A National Cholesterol Education Program (NCEP) Step II diet, containing 7 percent of the energy from SFAs, 25 percent from fat, 59 percent from CHOs, and 200 mg of cholesterol. (3) An olive oil diet (OO). (4) A peanut oil diet (PO). (5) A peanut and peanut butter diet (PPB). The last three diets contained a high percentage of polyunsaturated fatty acids.

The three high-MUFA diets (3, 4, and 5) contained the same amount of SFAs as the NCEP Step II diet. In these diets, however, some of CHO energy was exchanged for MUFA, but total fat in these diets was the same as in the AAD, which was 35 percent of total energy intake.

Plasma cholesterol levels were reduced in four diets in comparison with the AAD. On the NCEP Step II diet and PO diet, the subjects' plasma total cholesterol levels were reduced by 9 percent. Plasma total cholesterol levels were reduced by 11 percent on the OO diet, and PPB diet, from an average total cholesterol level of 209 mg/dl on the AAD diet. The LDL-cholesterol levels of the subjects were decreased by an average of 14 percent following all of the four diets compared with the AAD diet. The NCEP Step II diet caused an 11 percent increase in serum levels of triacylglycerol and a 4 percent decrease in HDL-cholesterol. In the three high-MUFA diets subjects decreased serum levels of triacylglycerols by 13 percent and showed no net change in HDL-cholesterol.

The investigators of this study, based on their findings, predicted that the OO diet may result in the largest reduction in the risk of cardiovascular diseases. The PPB diet and PO diet would be second and third in decreasing the risk respectively. They also concluded that a diet high in MUFAs is better than low-fat and high-carbohydrate diets in reducing the risk of cardiovascular diseases.[25]

CVDs Risk Factors Unrelated to Dietary Cholesterol

Risk factors for CVDs are many. These factors include genetics, lifestyle, obesity, diabetes, smoking, alcohol consumption, stressful living, high dietary fat and saturated fat, and lack of physical activity. In this chapter only a few of these risk factors are discussed.

Smoking

Data from a study of 106,745 middle-aged Korean men show that between 1990 and 1992 smoking was a great independent risk factor for stroke and atherosclerotic and cardiovascular diseases, especially ischemic heart disease. Follow-up studies over 6 years proved that smoking definitely increases the risk of stroke and other cardiovascular diseases in middle-aged Korean men with normal serum cholesterol levels.[26] Although smoking is mostly blamed for causing death due to cancer of the respiratory system, it is a recognized risk factor for CHD, stroke, hyperlipidemia, and atherosclerotic diseases.

Excess Body Weight

Excess body weight has been shown to be one of factors mostly associated with morbidity. Must et al. used the data from the third National Health Examination survey (NHANES III) to show the relationship of excess body weight and risk of coronary heart disease. These data showed that 65 percent of males and 55 percent of females in United States are overweight or obese. The data also showed that serum cholesterol levels are higher in the overweight and obese individuals than the people with normal weight. Serum levels of cholesterol did not increase proportionally with increases in weight. The conclusions reached by the investigators indicated that many of the degenerative disease such as hypertension, hypercholesterolemia, and coronary heart disease, among many others, are related to excess body weight.[27] Fine et al. showed that excess body weight and weight gain in women in the Nurses' Health Study were associated with a decrease in vitality and impaired physical function and pain while maintained or slightly decreased body weight was associated with more vitality and physical function and less pain. Distribution of excess fat throughout the body can also be a determinant of risk for CVDs. Upper abdomen fat accumulation is recognized as a risk factor.

Results of both studies indicated that good health and absence of disease are associated with normal body mass index (BMI) and maintaining normal weight. Normal BMI not only maintains health and physical function but it also is one way of reducing the risk of morbidity.[28]

LDL Oxidation

It is well established that circulating LDL-cholesterol when oxidized becomes a risk factor in cardiovascular diseases. Many studies have shown that a diet high in antioxidants can reduce the risk of cardiovascular diseases by preventing the oxidation of LDL-cholesterol. This is the basis of the recommendation for high intake of fruits and vegetables in the Dietary Guidelines for American Adults. Many fruits and vegetables are loaded with antioxidants such as β-carotene, vitamin C, α-tocopherol, and many phytochemicals that also have antioxidant activity. Anderson et al. investigated the effect of antioxidants on prevention of LDL oxidation in patients with type II diabetes and matched controls. The type II diabetic patients' diets were supplemented with 24 mg β-carotene, 1000 mg ascorbate, and 800 IU of α-tocopherol, while the control group received placebos. LDL oxidation rates were measured using four different techniques. The results showed that antioxidant supplementation is effective in reducing the rate of oxidation of LDL in type II diabetics.[29]

Level of Homocystein

The level of homocystein in the serum is believed to be one of the risk factors for coronary heart disease. Homocystein has an oxidant effect on LDL-C. Oxidized LDL-C initiates or compounds plaque formation in the arteries, causing atherosclerotic lesions. It is believed that elevated circulating levels of homocystein in serum, either severely or mildly, increases the risk of vascular occlusion. Brattstrom and Wilcken[30] discussed whether homocystein elevation in the serum is a cause of atherosclerotic vascular disease or result of the same. Chait and colleagues showed that by fortifying the diet of study subjects with histories of hypertension, dyslipidemia, type II diabetes, or combination of these diseases with 100 percent of the RDA for 23 micronutrients, plasma concentration of homocystein was decreased, reducing risk of coronary heart disease. They increased dietary intake of folate, vitamin B_6, and vitamin B_{12} by 399 μg/day, 7.4 μg/day, and 2.1 μg/day respectively in the study group over the amounts of these nutrients in the control diet. The results of the study showed that increasing the amount of these nutrients, which are cofactors in many metabolic pathways, in the diet of the study group lowered plasma homocystein concentrations effectively, decreasing LDL-C oxidation and the risk of coronary heart disease.[31]

Egg Consumption and Risk of Cardiovascular Diseases

Hu and colleagues studied a population of 117,000 individuals that included 80,082 women in the Nurses' Health Study who were followed for 14 years and 37,851 men in the Health Professionals follow-up study that were followed for 8 years. The study began in 1986 for men and in 1976 for women. Average egg consumption of participants was surveyed in 2-year intervals. The results showed that egg consumption declined in men from an average of 2.3 eggs/week in 1986 to 1.6 in 1990. In women consumption of eggs decreased from an average of 2.8/week in 1986 to 1.4 eggs/week in 1990. Those with higher egg consumption ate more foods high in dietary cholesterol and protein but consumed less low-fat food and fewer vegetables and fruits.

They also found that egg consumption was positively related to unhealthy eating habits, such as consumption of whole milk, red meat and bacon, high-fat foods, low level of exercise, and smoking, in men. When the data were adjusted for smoking and consumption of fatty foods and bacon, the relationship between egg consumption and CVDs became slightly inverse, indicating the lack of association between egg consumption and risk of CVDs. They also showed that egg consumption appeared to indicate risk of CVDs in a subgroup of subjects with diabetes.

Additionally they examined the data to see if any association could be found in consumption of eggs and risk of CVDs in other subgroups selected for hyperlipidemia, age, hypertension, smoking, alcohol use, body mass index, vitamin supplement intake, intake of SFAs, PUFAs, and carbohydrates, and family history of myocardial infarction (MI). They found no association between higher consumption of eggs in any of the subgroups and the risk of CVDs. Investigators found no significant relationship between consumption of eggs and rate of cardiovascular diseases in either men or women. "We specifically found no evidence for a significant increase in risk with either recent or relatively long-term (over the past decade) egg consumption. Despite somewhat different patterns of egg consumption in men and women, the results of the 2 cohorts were remarkably consistent." They found no difference in the risk of heart diseases between those who ate less than one egg per week and those who consumed more than one egg per day.[32] This study illustrates the importance of looking at the overall eating habits of individuals and takes into account subjects' health status and genetic background in relation to the effect of egg consumption on the risk of CVDs.

Reports of two meta-analysis studies on the effects of dietary fat and cholesterol on plasma lipids and lipoproteins were published in 1997. Clark et al. analyzed data from 82 metabolic ward studies.[8] Howell et al.[33] used results of 224 studies involving about 8,000 metabolic ward subjects. Howell's study included data from subjects with controlled feeding and also those who were free-living, with self-selected diets. Results from both studies are very similar and indicate that changing 1 percent of calories in saturated fatty acids to PUFAs lowers plasma total cholesterol by 3 mg/dl and LDL-cholesterol by 2.3 mg/dl. When dietary cholesterol is decreased by 50 mg/day total plasma cholesterol and LDL-cholesterol are lowered by 1 mg/dl. A decreased percentage of calories from fat replaced with carbohydrates results in lowered plasma HDL-cholesterol. They found that most of the studies published since 1990 gave predictive equations that indicate when dietary cholesterol is reduced 100 mg, plasma cholesterol is reduced by 35.43–69.3 μmol/L or 1.37 to 2.68 mg/dl. The result of the meta-analysis by Howell et al. predicts that plasma cholesterol response to reduction of 100 mg/day dietary cholesterol is a reduction of 56.9 μmol/l or 2.2 mg/dl. This is about a 1 percent decrease of plasma cholesterol concentration in an average population.

These results differ from the 1988 report of the National Institutes of Health workshop on the effect of dietary cholesterol on plasma cholesterol[34] suggesting that in a 4,185 kJ/day diet a 100 mg increase in dietary cholesterol will raise the plasma cholesterol levels by 259 μmol/l or 10 mg/day. This meta-analysis study showed that plasma LDL-cholesterol concentration is related to changes in dietary SFAs and PUFAs, but changes in plasma HDL-cholesterol concentrations are related to changes of dietary SFAs and total dietary fat.

Conner,[35] discussing the effect of cholesterol and different dietary saturated fatty acids on the incidence of coronary heart disease, held cholesterol less responsible for CHD due to the results of studies of recent years. He also indicated that fatty acids with less than 10 carbons are handled like carbohydrates by the body rather than fat, having no effect on the concentration of plasma cholesterol.

It has been shown that stearic acid with 18 carbon atoms is benign and does not elevate the blood cholesterol levels. After absorption and circulation by chylomicron and chylomicron remnants, it is picked up by the liver, and there it is changed into monounsaturated fatty acid by liver enzymes for its conversion to MUFA. Other investigators have shown that dietary stearic acid increases the risk of CHD more than the other saturated fatty acids.[36] Thus, Conner believed that the effect of stearic acid on increasing the risk of CHD may be due to its pathogenic effects before it is taken up by the liver and not after its conversion to oleic acid. It is known that dietary stearic acid decreases the HDL levels in the blood.[37] Stearic acid has also been shown to be thrombogenic by activating platelets and promoting coagulation.

The foods that promote death due to CHD are red meat, whole milk and dairy products made with whole milk, chocolate, lard, coconut oil, high-fat "fast foods," and highly hydrogenated margarines and shortenings (containing *trans*fatty acids). Interestingly, eggs are not listed among these foods. Also of interest is that whole milk group foods are highly associated with death due to CHD. The rate of death from CHD in Finland is five times that in other countries. Consumption of whole milk and its products is also much higher in Finland.[38] Missing from the above list of pathogenic foods other than eggs are some foods with very a high content of cholesterol. These foods include organ meats.

Sutherland and colleagues studied the effect of increasing the consumption of eggs on plasma cholesteryl esters transfer protein activity in healthy men and women. They found that increased consumption of eggs increased the plasma cholesterol levels in plasma apo B–containing lipoprotein (very low density lipoprotein–cholesterol + LDL-cholesterol) with no change in HDL levels. In women, however, little increase in apolipoprotein B fraction was observed while the HDL-cholesterol levels were increased. These investigators believed that decrease in the plasma newly synthesized cholesterol ester transfer (NCET) activity prevented increased apolipoprotein B cholesterol in response to increased cholesterol consumption in the women "by slowing the transfer of cholesteryl esters from HDL to lipoprotein containing apoB."[39] These investigators concluded that increased intake of cholesterol in the form of added eggs to the diet of free-living men and women consuming normal diets decreased the transfer of newly synthesized cholesteryl esters from HDL to atherogenic lipoproteins in plasma. This phenomenon happens more in older people, women, and those who habitually consume a diet high in cholesterol.

An increase in plasma cholesterol ester transfer protein (CETP) concentrations and activity is associated with predisposing the individual to atherosclerosis.[40] It has been shown that individuals who have a deficiency of this protein have a high level of plasma HDL-cholesterol and apolipoprotein A-I and a low risk for coronary heart disease.[41]

Jensen et al.[42] studied the effect of lipid-lowering diets on changes in plasma cholesterol ester transfer protein concentrations in young men. They used (1) a high saturated fatty acid diet containing 38 percent of calories as fat, 20 percent of which was saturated, (2) the National Cholesterol Education Program (NCEP) Diet Step I containing 28 percent fat, 10 percent saturated, and (3) a monounsaturated fatty acid–rich diet at 38 percent fat with 22 percent monounsaturated fatty acids. Forty-one healthy normolipidemic men participated in this study for three consecutive 4-week periods on each diet. Only the two lipid-lowering diets in this study (NCEP and MUSF) decreased plasma total and LDL-cholesterol, apo B, and CETP. The NCEP Step I diet decreased plasma HDL levels.

Investigators have shown that by reducing high-carbohydrate foods in the diet and adding eggs high-density lipoprotein cholesterol, which is commonly called good cholesterol, is elevated.[43] Stucchi et al. studied cholesterolemic response of cynomolgus monkeys to dietary cholesterol fed as egg yolks. The monkeys were fed diets containing 30 to 36 percent of daily calories as fat. They received a low-cholesterol (0.01 mg/Kj), medium cholesterol (0.03mg/Kj), and high-cholesterol diet (0.05 mg/Kj) in three different study periods lasting 30, 32, and 24 weeks respectively. They showed that serum total cholesterol, LDL-C, and LDL apolipoprotein B concentration were increased parallel with the level of dietary cholesterol. Serum HDL levels were not changed. They concluded that "cynomolgus monkeys are hyperresponsive to dietary cholesterol compared to humans, suggesting that this model may be useful in identifying metabolic and genetic predictors of hyperresponsiveness to dietary cholesterol in humans as well as assessing the metabolic heterogeneity of response to dietary cholesterol."[44]

Analysis of data from 24 countries show that there is a negative relationship between per capita egg consumption and incidence of cardiovascular mortality. Japan, France, and Spain are three of the highest–egg-consuming nations. Japan is the highest–egg-consuming nation with 6.3 eggs per person per week and the lowest rate of heart disease. The other two countries have the lowest incidence of cardiovascular mortality among the industrial nations. At this point a quote from Ancel Keys is appropriate: "there's no connection whatsoever between food and cholesterol in the blood. None. And we've known that all along."[45]

The fact that eggs keep bad company in the diet of the Western world cannot be overlooked. The usual breakfast menus list eggs with *bacon, sausage,* and *cheese,* usually consumed with toast and *butter* or other high–saturated fat foods such as red meat.[46] This breakfast is usually followed by a lunch consisting of fast foods (hamburgers and fries, tacos, fried chicken, or hot dogs). The dinner menu usually contains one type of meat plus other fatty foods and rich deserts. This type of unhealthy diet is definitely the best way to increase the risk of CVDs in susceptible individuals. The cholesterol content of eggs in this diet is only a small fraction of the total cholesterol in the diet. Saturated fat alone in the diet is an important risk factor for CVDs.

The types of dietary practices that the majority of Americans indulge in have been the reason health professionals resist changing the recommendation to restrict eggs to not more that three to four per week. However, it is not certain that this recommendation will discourage people to decrease their consumption of foods high in saturated fat. Messages from health professionals and health organizations alerting people about the dangers of foods high in saturated fats are abundant. Unfortunately, these health messages are ignored by the majority of people. Dietary fat consumption has not decreased significantly, in spite of all the recommendations to reduce dietary fat intake to 30 percent of daily energy intake and saturated fat intake to less than 10 percent. People continue consuming their high-fat diets, frequenting fast food establishments, and eating high-fat meats, dairy products, and rich deserts.

Egg Alternatives and New Eggs in the Market

Egg alternatives have been suggested by health professionals and have appeared in the market for years. These egg alternatives have been used by people who, for reasons of health, could not consume eggs. Egg Beaters, which is mostly egg white with vegetable oil, flavor, and color to simulate the yolk, is one product that has been used successfully by people. It has been recommended to use two egg whites in place of one egg in recipes. This practice has been very popular among those who have a high plasma cholesterol levels and cannot eat eggs.

Newly developed eggs with lower fats and cholesterol are one of the efforts by the food industry to satisfy the appetite of egg-loving people without jeopardizing their health. Egg industry researchers now have developed a few different eggs by feeding hens special diets. For example, researchers, knowing that flaxseed is very rich in omega-3 fatty acids such as docosahexanoic acid (DHA), also found in fatty fish, fed it to hens. DHA was recovered from the yolks of the eggs from hens that ate a flaxseed diet.

Another type of designer egg with enriched nutrients on the supermarket shelf now is Gold Circle Farm Eggs. This egg contains 750 percent more DHA, vitamin B_{12} in this egg is increased 300 percent, and vitamin E 600 percent.[47] Eggstasy is a designer egg developed, patented, and produced by the University of Wisconsin. This egg has 25 percent less fat, a total of 3.5 g per egg, 17 percent less cholesterol at 180 mg, and 300 percent more vitamin E. Egglands Best was the first egg that was developed by feeding hens a specially modified diet to reduce fat and cholesterol and modify the type of fatty acids in the yolk.

Surai et al., in a double-blind placebo-controlled study in which 40 healthy adult subjects were matched for age and sex, evaluated designer eggs enriched with vitamin E, lutein, selenium, and DHA. DHA is an omega-3 fatty acid that lowers LDL-C and prevents platelet aggregation, lowering the risk of CHD. They showed that subjects on the designer eggs diet significantly increased in plasma levels of DHA, lutein, and α-tocopherol in comparison with subjects consuming normal eggs. In this study the largest increase was found in lutein, with a 1.88-fold increase. "The proportion of DHA was increased in all the main lipid classes of the plasma including triacylglycerol (2-, 3-fold), free fatty acids (1.6-fold), cholesteryl ester (1.4-fold) and phospholipids (1.3-fold)." The concentration of selenium in plasma, blood pressure, total plasma lipid concentration, and concentration of total cholesterol and HDL-cholesterol in plasma did not change.[48]

This study proves that designer foods with altered nutrients much better suited for healthy eating can provide an alternative for those people who for genetic or other reasons should not eat regular eggs. This includes people who are hypersensitive to dietary cholesterol—their plasma levels of cholesterol respond to dietary cholesterol and are susceptible to cardiovascular diseases. It must be kept in mind that only a small percentage of people are among this group. The rest of the population can enjoy eggs provided they use prudence in choosing other foods and practice healthy eating habits.

References

1. Food and Agriculture Organization of the United Nations. The Amino Acid Content of Foods and Biological Data on Proteins. Nutritional Study #24. Rome, 1970.
2. Food and Agriculture Organization of the United Nations, The Amino Acid Content of Foods and Biological Data on Proteins. Nutritional Study #24. Rome, 1970.
3. Evenepoel, P., Geypens, B., Luypaerts, A., Hiele, M., and Ghoos, Y. Digestibility of cooked and raw egg protein in humans as assessed by stable isotope techniques. J Nutr 1998;128:1716–22.
4. 1989 Supplement-Agriculture Handbook No. 8. Human Nutrition Information Service, USDA.
5. National Cholesterol Education Program. Report of the expert panel on population strategies for blood cholesterol reduction: executive summary. Arch Intern Med 1991;151:1071–84.
6. Hegsted, D.M., McGandy, R.B., Myers, M.L., and Stare F.J. Quantitative effect of dietary fat on serum cholesterol in man. Am J Clin Nutr 1965;17:281–95.
7. Keys, A., and Parlin, R.W. Serum cholesterol response to changes in dietary lipids. Am J Clin Nutr 1966;19:175–81.
8. Clark, R., Frost, C., Collins, R., Appleby, P., and Peto, R. Dietary lipids and blood cholesterol: quantitative meta analysis of metabolic wards studies. BMJ 1997;314:112–17.
9. McNamara, D.J. Cholesterol intake and plasma cholesterol: an update. J Am Coll Nutr 1997;16:530–34.
10. Block, G., Dresser, C.M., Hartman, A.M., and Carrell, M.D. Nutrient sources in the American diet: quantitative data from the NHANES II survey. II. Macronutrients and fats. Am J Epidemiol 1985;122:27–40.
11. Anderson, K.M., Wilson, P.W.F., Odell, P.M., and Kannel, W.B. In Cholesterol and Coronary Heart Disease, Gold, P., Grover, S., and Roncari, D.A.K., eds. Park Ridge: Patthenon, 1992, pp. 3–17.
12. Goodman, D.S. Report of the national cholesterol program expert panel on detection, evaluation, and treatment of high blood cholesterol in adults. Arch Intern Med 1988;148:36–68.
13. Newman, W.P., III, Freemand, D.S., Voors, A.W., Grad, P.D., Srinivasan, S.R., Cresanta, J.L., Williamson, G.D., Webber, L.S., and Berensen, G.S. Relation of serum lipoprotein levels and systolic blood pressure to early arteriosclerosis. N Engl J Med 1986;314:138–44.
14. Hegsted, D.M. Unanswered questions. In Proceedings from the Conference on the Effects of Dietary Fatty Acids on Serum Lipoproteins and Homeostasis, Nicolosi, R.J., ed. Washington DC: American Heart Association, 1989, pp. 103–14.
15. Keys, A., Anderson, J.T., and Grande, F. Serum cholesterol response to dietary fat. Lancet 1957;1:787.
16. Mattson, F.H., Erickson, B.A., and Klingman, A.M. Effect of dietary cholesterol on serum cholesterol in man. Am J Clin Nutr 1972;25:589–94.
17. Schonfeld, G., Patsch, W., Rudel, L.L., Nelson, C., Epstein, M., and Olsen, R.E. Effects of

dietary cholesterol and fatty acids on plasma lipoproteins. J Clin Invest 1982;69:1072–80.

18. Martin, L.J., Connelly, P.W., Manco, D., Woods, N.S., Zhang, Z.J., Mguire, G., Quinet, E., Tall, A.R., Marcel, Y.A., McPherson, R. Cholesteryl ester transfer protein and response to cholesterol feeding in men. Relationship to apo protein E genotype. J Lipid Res 1993;34:437–46.
19. Clifton, P.M., Abbey, M., Noakes, M., Beltrame, S., Rumbllow, N., and Nestel, P. Body fat distribution is a determinant of the high-density lipoprotein response to dietary cholesterol in women. Arteroscler Thromp Vasc Biol 1995;15:1070–78.
20. Havel, R.J. Functional activities of hepatic lipoprotein receptors. Ann Rev Physiol 1986;48:119–34.
21. Stange, E.F., and Dietschy, J.M. Cholesterol absorption and metabolism by the intestinal epithelium. In New Comprehensive Biochemistry: Sterols and Bile Acids, vol. 12, Danielsson, H., and Sjovall, J. eds. Netherlands: Elsevier Science, 1985, pp. 121–49.
22. Nervi, F.O., Weis, H.J., and Dietschy, J.M. The kinetic characteristics of inhibition of hepatic cholesterogenesis by lipoproteins of intestinal origin. J Biol Chem 1975;250:4145–51.
23. Fielding, C.J. Factors affecting the rate of catalyzed transfer of cholesteryl esters in plasma. Am Heart J 1987;113:532–37.
24. Spady, D.K., Woollett, L.A., and Dietschy, J.M. Regulation of plasma LDL-cholesterol levels by dietary cholesterol and fatty acids. Ann Rev Nutr 1993;13:355–81.
25. Kris-Etherton, P.M., Pearson, T.A., Wan, Y., Hargrove, R.L., Moriarity, K., Fishell, V., and Etherton, T.D. High monounsaturated fatty acid diets lower both plasma cholesterol and triacylglycerol concentrations. Am J Clin Nutr 1999;70:1009–15.
26. Jee, S.H., Suh, I., Kim, I.S., and Appel, L.J. Smoking and atherosclerotic cardiovascular disease in men with low levels of serum cholesterol. JAMA 1999;282:2149–55.
27. Must, A., Spadano, J., Coakley, E.H., Field, A.E., Coldtz, G., and Dietz, W.J. The disease burden associated with overweight and obesity. JAMA 1999;282:1523–29.
28. Fine, J.T., Colditz, G.A., Coakley, E.H., Moseley, Manson, J.E., Willett, W.C., and Kawachi, L. A prospective study of weight change and health-related quality of life in women. JAMA 1999;282:2136–42.
29. Anderson, J.W., Gowri, M.S., Turner, J., Nichols, L., Diwadkar, V.A., Chow, C.K., and Oeltgen, P.R. Antioxidant supplementation effects on low-density lipoprotein oxidation for individuals with type-2 diabetes mellitus. J Am Coll Nutr 1999;18:451–61.
30. Brattstrom, L., and Wilcken, E.L. Homocystein and cardiovascular disease: cause and effect. Am J Clin Nutr 2000;72:315-23.
31. Chait, A., Malinow, M.R., and Morris, C.D. Increased dietary micronutrients decrease serum homocystein concentrations in patients at high risk of cardiovascular disease. Am J Clin Nutr 1999;70:881–87.
32. Hu, F.B., Stampfer, M.J., Rimm, E.B., Manson, J.E., Ascherio, A., Colditz, G.A., Rosner, B.A., Spiegelman, D., Speizer, F.E., Sacks, F.M., Hennekens, C.H., and Willett, W.C. A prospective study of egg consumption and risk of cardiovascular disease in men and women. JAMA 1999;281:1387–94.
33. Howell, W.H., McNamara, D.J., Tosca, M.A., Smith, B.T., and Gains, J.A. Plasma lipid and lipoprotein response to dietary fat and cholesterol: a meta-analysis. Am J Clin Nutr 1997;65:1747-64.
34. Grundy, S.M., Barrett-Conner, E., Rudel, L.L., Mietten, T., and Spector, A.A. Workshop on the impact of dietary cholesterol on plasma lipoproteins and atherogenesis. Atherosclerosis 1988;8:95–101.

35. Conner, W.E. Harbingers of coronary heart disease: dietary saturated fatty acids and cholesterol. Is chocolate benign because of its stearic acid content? Am J Clin Nutr 1999;70:951–52.
36. Hu, F.B., Stampfer, M.J., Manson, J.E., Ascherio, A., Couitz, G.A., Speizer, F.E., Hennekens, C.H., and Willett, W.C. Dietary saturated fats and their food sources in relation to the risk of coronary heart disease in women. Am J Clin Nutr 1999;70:1001–8.
37. Aro, A. Jauhiainen, Mpartanen, R., Salminen, L., and Mutanen, M. Stearic acid, trans fatty acids and dietary fat: effects on serum and lipoprotein lipids, apolipoproteins, lipoprotein (a), and lipid transfer proteins in healthy subjects. Am J Clin Nutr 1997;65:1419–26.
38. Artoud-Wild, S.M., Conner, S.L., Sexton, G., and Conner, W.E. Differences in coronary mortality can be explained by differences in cholesterol and saturated fat intakes in forty countries but not in France and Finland. Circulation 1993;88:2771–79.
39. Sutherland, W.H.F., Ball, M.J., and Walker, H. The effect of increased egg consumption on plasma cholesteryl ester transfer activity in healthy subjects. Eur J Clin Nutr 1997;51:172–76.
40. Bagdade, J.D., Ritter, M.C., and Subbaiah, P.V. Accelerated cholesterol ester transfer in patients with insulin dependant diabetes mellitus. Eur J Clin Nutr 1991;21:162–67.
41. Koizumi, J., Inazu, A., Kunimas, Y., Yagi, K., Koizumi, I., Uno, Y., Kajinami, K., Miyamoto, S., Moulin, P., and Maabuct, I.H. Serum lipoprotein lipids concentration and composition in homozygous and heterozygous patients with cholesteryl ester transfer protein deficiency. Atherosclerosis 1991;90:189–96.
42. Jensen, S., Lopez-Miranda, J., Castro, P., Lopez-Segurd, F., Marin, C., Ordoras, J.M., Jimenez-pereperez, J., Fuentes, F., and Perz-Jimenes, F. Low-fat and hi-monounsaturated fatty acid diets decrease plasma cholesterol ester transfer protein concentrations in young, healthy normolipemic men. Am J Clin Nutr 2000;72:36–41.
43. Schnohr, P., Thomson, O., Riis Hanson, P., Boberg, Ans, G., Lawaetz, H., and Weeke, T. Egg consumption and high density lipoprotein cholesterol. J Intern Med 1994;23:249–51.
44. Stucchi, A.F., Nicolosi, R.J., and Karge, W.H., III, Ausman, L.M., and Ordovas, J.M. Dietary cholesterol affects serum lipoproteins and LDL metabolism in cynomolgus monkeys in a dose-response manner. J Nutr 1998;128:1104–13.
45. Keys, A. Eating Well. March/April 1997 issue.
46. Krauss, R.M., Deckelbaum, R.J., Ernst, N., Fisher, E., Howerd, B.V., Knopp, R.H., Kotchen, T., Lichtenstein, A.H., McGill, H.C., Pearson, T.A., Prewitt, T.E., Stone, N.J., VanHorn, L., and Weinberg, R. Dietary guidelines for healthy american adults, a statement for health professionals from the Nutrition Committee, American Heart Association. Circulation 1996;94:1795–1800.
47. Gold Circle Farms Eggs, Newsletter, 2000, http//www.goldcirclefarms.com/info.htm.
48. Surai, P.F., MacPherson, A., Speake, B.K., and Speaks, N.H.C. Designer egg evaluation in a controlled trial. Eur J Clin Nutr 2000;54:298–305.

10

Effect of Dietary Eggs on Human Serum Cholesterol and Coronary Heart Disease

Yinhong Chen
and Ronald R. Watson

INTRODUCTION

Eggs contain cholesterol in 372 to 444 mg/100 g of the consumable portion. Most people regard the amount of eggs in their diets as a significant factor in increasing serum cholesterol and as a risk factor for coronary heart disease (CHD). Recommendations of dietary restriction of eggs to prevent high serum cholesterol and CHD have been widely accepted. However, many researchers challenge this hypothesis due to insufficient evidence and multifactorial etiology CHD. Egg consumption could be a factor contributing to high serum cholesterol levels especially in individuals with genetic defects, but evidence, though insufficient, suggests the presence of other possible risk factors is required for deleterious effects to become evident. Thus, because findings are inconsistent, the egg cholesterol–CHD hypothesis may be premature. Eggs are rich sources of protein, have essential amino acids and vitamins that are readily available, and are inexpensive. Reevaluation of egg intake restriction is necessary.

Coronary heart disease is increasing at an alarming rate, becoming the number one killer in the Western world. However, it is no longer confined to Western Europe and the United States. CHD has spread throughout the world as people's lifestyles and eating habits have become more "westernized." Serum cholesterol level was determined to be one of the major risk factors for CHD because evidence exists that early atherosclerotic plaque consists of foam cell macrophages loaded with cholesterol, which is derived from the cellular uptake of oxidatively modified low-density lipoprotein (LDL). Dietary habits are significant influences on serum cholesterol levels.

Egg yolks are one of the richest sources of dietary cholesterol (Table 10.1). One egg contains about 200 mg of cholesterol. In recent years, the total consumption of eggs has declined appreciably. One reason is the belief that the yolk's high cholesterol concentration is unhealthy. The American Heart Association and Surgeon General have both recommended restricting dietary cholesterol to 300 mg per day.[1] The National Cholesterol Education Program (NCEP) guidelines recommend dietary restriction of fat and cholesterol to reduce high circulating cholesterol concentrations in adult Americans. The recommendation that no more than 300 mg cholesterol be consumed daily to prevent a high serum cholesterol level and CHD is often used to justify a restriction of egg intake to three or four per week.

However, much clinical and epidemiological data[2–6] demonstrate that dietary cholesterol has little effect on plasma cholesterol in most individuals. Cholesterol is not an activator but an indicator of the arteriosclerotic process taking place within the vascular wall; in fact, a chronic inflammation is the strongest predictor of CHD. Thus, researchers have raised a number of questions regarding the justification of population-wide restrictions on egg consumption in the last decade.

Egg Cholesterol Content

Ingr et al. reported that egg cholesterol content varied from 1,200 to 1,360 mg/100 g of yolk or from 372 to 444 mg/100 g of the consumable portion of the egg. Through the egg-laying period, the yolk cholesterol content fluctuated rather irregularly and showed great variability with a variation coefficient of 9.7–18.2 percent.[8] Significant differences in cholesterol concentrations were found by Barir and Marion between domestic and wild genetic groups of turkeys and ducks. Species listed in increasing concentration of cholesterol per gram of yolk were guinea fowl, chicken, pheasant, quail, turkey, duck, goose, and dove, with an overall range of 12.77 to 21.99 mg of cholesterol per gram of yolk.[9] It was also found that yolk cholesterol tended to decrease as the hen's age increased. Due to eco-

Table 10.1. Egg contents

One egg	Weight (g)	Fat (g)	SFA (g)	UFA (g)	PUFA (g)	Cholesterol (mg)
Chicken egg						
Boiled egg	50	5.3	1.6	2.0	0.7	212
Fried egg	46	6.9	1.9	2.7	1.3	211
Poached egg	50	5.0	1.5	1.9	0.7	212
Dried egg	5	2.2	0.7	0.9	0.3	101
Fresh/frozen egg	50	5.0	1.6	1.9	0.7	213
Egg yolk	17	5.2	1.6	2.0	0.7	218
Egg white	33	0.0	0.0	0.0	0.0	0
Duck egg	70	9.6	2.6	4.6	0.9	619
Goose egg	144	19.1	5.2	8.3	2.4	1227
Turkey egg	79	9.4	2.9	3.6	1.3	737

Source. Modified from Reference 7.
Note. SFA = saturated fatty acid, UFA = unsaturated fatty acid, and PUFA = polyunsaturated fatty acid.

nomics or other conditions, intensive market egg production was found to be associated with a decrease in yolk cholesterol content because of practices such as using cholesterol biosynthesis enzyme inhibitors in laying hens, creating genetic hybrids in different strains of hens, and altering the fatty acid composition of yolk lipids through manipulation of laying hens' diets.[10,11–13] Thus, the properties of chicken eggs could be modified in favorable ways.

Cholesterol Metabolism

Cholesterol is a four-ring hydrocarbon with an eight-carbon side. It is either absorbed from the diet or synthesized by cells in the body. In humans, about 10–20 percent of total cholesterol synthesis occurs in the liver.

After a cholesterol-rich meal, cholesterol and triglycerides (TGs) are absorbed into the mucosal cells of the small intestine as free cholesterol. There they are esterified to cholesteryl esters and packaged with apo B-48, apo A-2, and apo A-4 into chylomicrons and released into the blood via the lymphatic system. The chylomicron particle acquires apo E and apo C-2/C-3 in lymph and plasma. In capillary beds, TG is hydrolyzed by lipoprotein lipase (LPL). When chylomicrons are hydrolyzed by the LPL, their surface coating unesterifies cholesterol. The remnant particle is then removed primarily by the liver, mediated by binding to low-density lipoprotein receptor–related protein (LRP) and low-density lipoprotein receptor (LDLR) as well as to surface proteoglycans. Significant dietary cholesterol is also transferred into high-density lipoprotein (HDL) particles mediated by cholesterol ester transfer protein (CETP). HDL accepts unesterified cholesterol associated with lecithin-cholesterol acyltransferase (LCAT) to produce cholesteryl ester. The HDL particle with cholesteryl ester is transported to the liver by SR-B1 receptors. In addition, very low-density lipoprotein (VLDL), intermediate-density lipoprotein (IDL), or LDL can return cholesterol esters to the liver indirectly via CETP. This HDL/LCAT/CETP system plays a pivotal role in removing excess cellular cholesterol, facilitating its transfer back to the liver for excretion.

Endogenous cholesterol synthesis begins with acetate. Three acetate molecules are condensed to form 3-hydroxy-3-methylglutaryl-coenzyme A (HMG-CoA), which is then converted into mevalonic acid by the enzyme HMG-CoA reductase. The key (rate-limiting) step regulating cholesterol biosynthesis involves HMG-CoA reductase. Increased cholesterol content of cells feeds back on the HMG-CoA reductase, decreases its activity, and thereby decreases cholesterol biosynthesis. Conversely, a deficiency of intracellular cholesterol increases reductase activity and increases cholesterol biosynthesis. Cholesterol cannot be eliminated by catabolism to carbon dioxide and water; it must be either excreted as free cholesterol in the bile or converted to bile acids and secreted into the intestine. The conversion of cholesterol to bile acids accounts for approximately 70 percent of the cholesterol disposed of daily.[14] Cholesterol levels in the blood are controlled primarily through the LDL receptor pathway. This receptor is present on the surface of all cells throughout the body. Specific proteins on the surface of certain lipoproteins (apolipoprotein B100 and apolipoprotein E) interact with the LDL receptor and facilitate lipoprotein internalization by cells. The number of LDL receptors on the cell surface is tightly regulated. If serum cholesterol is elevated, there is an increase in the number of receptors synthesized. The removal of excess cholesterol from arterial wall cells by HDL could play a crucial role in minimizing cholesterol accumulation in the artery wall and inhibiting atherogenesis.

Egg Intake and Serum Cholesterol Level

Epidemiological studies on the relationship of egg consumption to serum cholesterol level are sparse, and the results of such studies are inconsistent. These conflicting results have many possible explanations. One practical result of this interpretation has been the recommendation to limit egg consumption. However, many researchers challenge this theory.

Most people are concerned that the high cholesterol in eggs is unfavorable for health. Modified eggs or egg substitutes, which have low fat and cholesterol content, are now being researched. Several metabolic studies have suggested a hypocholesterolemic effect of decholesterolized eggs on blood cholesterol levels compared with whole eggs.[15,16] A study[17] revealed that modified eggs successfully reduced total serum levels of LDL- and HDL-cholesterol in subjects who ate 12 modified eggs over 6 weeks. Robert et al.[18] reported a study that compared the intake by outpatients of cholesterol-free egg substitutes and whole eggs. The mean plasma cholesterol level in the egg substitute group was not different from the baseline. The mean plasma cholesterol level in the whole egg group increased 9 percent above baseline level and 11 percent above the egg substitute group. Asato[19] found that consuming egg whites was associated with a favorable decrease in the total cholesterol and promoted a greater increase in HDL-cholesterol.

Many studies[3–6,20–22] reported that dietary cholesterol is not a significant factor in an individual's plasma cholesterol level. Reports from the Lipid Research Clinic's Research Prevalence Study and the Framingham Heart Study have also shown that dietary cholesterol is not related to either blood cholesterol or heart disease deaths. Many clinical trials[20–22] found that the addition of an egg or two a day to a low-fat diet has little if any effect on blood cholesterol levels. One hundred sixteen male volunteers between the ages of 32 and 62 consumed two whole fresh eggs daily in their customary diets for 3 months and also eliminated eggs from their diets for 3 months. No significant increase in mean serum cholesterol was found, nor was there a significant association of dietary cholesterol intake with serum cholesterol.[21] Vorster et al.[22] examined 70 young men who ate either 7 or 14 eggs a week for 5 months. Except for increased lecithin-cholesterol acyltransferase activities and total serum protein concentration, no significant differences in cholesterol were found. They also reported[23,24] that rural blacks that worked on an egg farm could handle a very high cholesterol intake (1,240 mg/day) without meaningful disturbance in serum HDL-, LDL-, and VLDL-cholesterol fractions. These findings suggested that researchers should probably concentrate on a reduction in fat and not cholesterol.

Some studies show that egg consumption differently increased composition of serum cholesterol level. Beynen and Katan[25] found that egg yolk consumption increased HDL by 36 percent and LDL by 21 percent. The HDL and LDL ratio increased by 16 percent. VLDL- and LDL-cholesterol decreased by 19 percent and 11 percent. Flynn et al. found[26] a significant increase of HDL in subjects eating three eggs daily for 10 weeks. However, the results are also inconsistent. Katan et al.[27] reported that egg yolk caused an unfavorable decrease in the mean ratio of HDL to total serum cholesterol. An increase in HDL may have been due to different fat intake with egg consumption in those subjects according to Jacotot et al.[28] They stated that the substitution of saturated with polyunsaturated fatty acid results in a reduction of total cholesterol, LDL-cholesterol, and HDL-cholesterol; the substitution of saturated with monounsaturated fatty acids reduces LDL-cholesterol without changing HDL-cholesterol; and the substitution of polyunsaturated with monounsaturated fatty acids has minimal effects on LDL-cholesterol but increases HDL-cholesterol.

Effect of Dietary Factors and Egg Intake on Serum Cholesterol Level

Dietary factors interfered with serum cholesterol levels when subjects concomitantly ate eggs. In one study,[29] healthy young men ate three eggs and 2 g of ascorbic acid a day, significantly increasing their total cholesterol and LDL-cholesterol. A possible synergistic relationship between these two dietary factors was suggested. Altering the fatty acid composition in diets also affected serum cholesterol levels in individuals who consumed eggs,[27,28,30] which confirmed Alberich and Motta's[28] theory. The complex interactions between various dietary lipids and components suggest that a single measure of fat intake is inadequate to assess the serum cholesterol level.

Individual Responses to Egg Intake in Serum Cholesterol Levels

Individual differences are attributed to an additional factor complicating the relationship between egg intake and serum cholesterol. Several reports[27,31] supported the existence of hypo- and hyperresponders to dietary cholesterol. The hyperresponders may have more efficient intestinal absorption of cholesterol and/or a defect of LDL receptor activity. The mechanism involved in suppressing cellular LDL receptor synthesis may be a major influence on increasing plasma LDL levels.[32] Extreme hyperresponders are individuals with familial homozygous hypercholesterolemia (1 in 1 million people) due to the absence of LDL receptors, resulting in a decreased capacity to remove plasma LDL. The plasma LDL levels may increase 6- to 10–fold. Heterozygous familial hypercholesterolemia has an even higher incidence in the population (1 in 500 individuals). These people demonstrate no receptors or produce abnormal nonfunctional LDL receptors with an approximated 2- to 3-fold increase in plasma LDL. In familial defective apolipoprotein B, the ligand-binding domain of apo B is defective because of a missense mutation at amino acid 3500. This mutation leads to impaired binding of the LDL to the LDL receptor and thus to clinical consequences of high plasma cholesterol level.

Interestingly, one hyporesponder[14] ate 25 eggs a day for many years and was almost completely free from clinical atherosclerosis and had normal plasma cholesterol. He ingested approximately 12,953 μmol of cholesterol a day, and 10,622 μmol passed through the patient's gastrointestinal tract to be excreted in the feces. He compensated further by doubling the usual rate of bile acid synthesis. Individual differences in response to diets suggested the operation of variables other than dietary factors, for instance, genetic factors, on serum cholesterol.

Egg Intake and CHD

Numerous papers[3–6,14,20–23,34–36] reported the relationship between diet and CHD. There is a controversy about the effect of dietary cholesterol on the concentration of serum cholesterol in humans. The inconsistencies in emerging studies comparing dietary cholesterol and CHD may be partly due to the complex interaction between dietary factors and serum cholesterol level. Some of the conflicting results are contributed to poor design. Some of them are due to individual differences in the sensitivity of serum cholesterol to dietary intake. Or researchers may have ignored the presence of other multirisk factors that are more important than high serum cholesterol in CHD. Hu et al.[3] reported that consumption of up to one egg per day is unlikely to have substantial overall impact on the risk of CHD among healthy men and women. However, an apparent increased risk of CHD associated with higher egg consumption was discovered among diabetic subjects. The increased risk may be related to abnormal cholesterol transport due to decreased levels of apolipoprotein E[33] and increased levels of apolipoprotein C-III.[34] The etiology of CHD is multifactorial. Egg consumption could be a factor in high serum cholesterol but not sufficient for development of CHD. CHD requires the presence of other possible risk factors for high serum cholesterol effects to become evident.

Egg Intake, Serum Cholesterol, and CHD

Even though the cause-and-effect relationship between hypercholesterolemia and CHD has been proven in a large number of animal model studies, in which reduced LDL-cholesterol levels dramatically reduced the risk of subsequent clinical CHD, the relationship between egg intake and cholesterol level can be challenged on the basis of human studies. The results are inconsistent, with some studies finding a positive relationship but some studies revealing no relationship between egg intake and cholesterol level.[3-6,20–23,35] Cliff[36] pointed out that "the daily intake of cholesterol was stupendously out of proportion to any sort of human dietary intake, equivalent to the consumption of approximately 110 eggs daily." Furthermore, the etiology of CHD is multifactorial. Schoefl[37] argued that lipids are not activators but indicators of the arteriosclerotic process taking place within the vascular wall. Hansson and Frostegard et al.[38,39] found a substantial proportion of activated T lymphocytes in carotid plaque specimens, the activation pattern of which was similar to that occurring under chronic inflammatory conditions. Moss[39] confirmed that inflammation was the strongest predictor of stenosis, while cholesterol was not significantly related to the degree of stenosis. If egg intake–increased serum cholesterol level contributes to a high incidence of CHD, the presence of other possible risk factors is also required for deleterious effects to become evident.

Eggs are readily available and inexpensive. Eggs are rich sources of protein, all the essential amino acids, thiamine, riboflavin, pantothenic and folic acid, vitamin B_{12}, biotin, vitamin D_3, vitamin E, and phosphorous. The relationships among egg intake, serum cholesterol, and CHD are inconsistent. These conflicting results could be attributed to other extraneous factors. Refined theories and research designed to resolve these inconsistencies are required. Before making a decision to restrict egg intake especially in a healthy person, we should individually evaluate the advantages and disadvantages of eating eggs. Recommendations should be based on overall nutritive content, not on cholesterol content alone.

References

1. Fairfield, P.B. The food and drug administration looks at cholesterol. J Assoc Food Drug Off 1991;55:41–44.
2. Vorster, H.H., Benade, A.J., Barnard, H.C., Locke, M.M., Silvis, N., Venter, C.S., Smuts, C.M., Engelbrecht, G.P., and Marais, M.P. Egg intake does not change plasma lipoprotein and coagulation profiles. Am J Clin Nutr 1992;55(2):400–10.
3. Hu, F.B., Stampfer, M.J., Rimm, E.B., Manson, J.E., Ascherio, A., Colditz, G.A., Rosner, B.A., Spiegelman, D., Speizer, F.E., Sacks, F.M., Hennekens, C.H., Willett, and W.C. A prospective study of egg consumption and risk of cardiovascular disease in men and women. JAMA 1999;281(15):1387–94.
4. Bronner, L.L., Kanter, D.S., and Manson, J.E. Primary prevention of stroke. N Engl J M 1995;333(21):1392–1400.
5. Bernstein, V., Cuddy, T.E., Moye, L.A., Piller, L.B., Rutherford, J., Simpson, L.M., and Braunwald, E. Reduction of stroke incidence after myocardial infarction with pravastatin: the Cholesterol and Recurrent Events (CARE) study. The CARE investigators. Circulation 1999;99(2):216–23.
6. Gillman, M.W., Cupples, L.A., Millen, B.E., Ellison, R.C., and Wolf, P.A. Inverse association of dietary fat with development of ischemic stroke in men. JAMA 1997;278(24):2145–50.
7. Pennington, J.A.T. Food Values of Portions Commonly Used. Seventeenth edition. Philadelphia; New York: Lippincott-Raven, 1998, pp. 73–74.
8. Ingr, I., Simeonova, J., Stavkova, J., Petrovshy, E., and Dostal, F. Cholesterol content in market hen eggs. Nahrung 1987;31(10):933–40.
9. Barir, C.W., and Marion, W.W. Yolk cholesterol in egg from various avian species. Poult Sci 1978;57(5):1260–65.
10. Elkin, R.G., Yan, Z., Zhong, Y., Donkin, S.S., Buhman, K.K., Story, J.A., Turek, J.J., Porter, R.E., Jr., Anderson, M., Homan, R., Newton, R.S. Select 3-hydroxy-3-methyglutary-coenzyme

A reductase inhibitors vary in their ability to reduce egg yolk cholesterol levels in laying hens through alteration of hepatic cholesterol biosynthesis and plasma VLDL composition. J Nutr 1999;129(5):1010–19.

11. Hood, R.L., Bailey, W.M., and Svoronos, D. The effect of dietary monterpenes on the cholestrol level of eggs. Poult Sci 1978;59(1):304–6.
12. Mori, A.V., Mendonca, C.X., Jr., and Santos, C.O. Effect of dietary lipid-lowering drugs upon plasma lipids and egg yolk cholesterol level of laying hens. J Agric Food Chem 1999;47(11):4731–35.
13. Kovacs, G., Dublecz, K., Husveth, F., Wagner, L., Gerendai, D., Orban, J., and Manilla, H. Effects of different hybrids, strains and age of laying hens on the cholesterol content of the table egg. Acta Vet Hung 1998;46(2):285–94.
14. Kern, Fred, Jr. Normal plasma cholesterol in a man who eats 25 eggs a day. N Engl J Med 1991;325(8):584.
15. Roberts, S.L., McMurry, M.P., and Connor, W.E. Does egg feeding (i.e., dietary cholesterol) affect plasma cholesterol levels in humans? The results of a double-blind study. Am J Clin Nutr 1981;34(10):2092–99.
16. Ginsberg, H.N., Karmally, W., Siddiqui, M., Holleran, S., Tall, A.R., Rumsey, S.C., Deckelbaum, R.J., Blaner, W.S., and Ramakrishnan, R. A dose-response study of the effects of dietary cholesterol on fasting and postprandial lipid and lipoprotein metabolism in healthy young men. Arteriosclerosis Thrombosis 1994;14(4):576–86.
17. Garwin, J.L., Organ, J., Stowell, R.L., Richardson, M.P., Walker, M.C., and Capuzzi, D. Modified eggs are compatible with a diet that reduces serum cholesterol concentration in humans. J Nutr 1992;122(11):2153–60.
18. Robert, S.L., Mcmurry, M.P., and Connor, W.E. Does egg feeding affect plasma cholesterol level in humans? The results of a double-blind study. Am J Clin Nutr 1981;34(10):2092–99.
19. Asato, L., Wang, M.F., Chan, Y.C., Yeh, S.H., Chung, H.M, Chung, S.Y., Chida, S., Uezato, T., Suzuki, I., and Yamagata, N. Effect of egg white on serum cholesterol concentration in young women. J Nutr Sci Vitaminol 1996;42:87–96.
20. Chenoweth, W., Ullmann, M., Simpson, R., and Leveille, G. Influence of dietary cholesterol and fat on serum lipids in men. J Nutr 1981;111(12):2069–80.
21. Flynn, M.A., Nolph, G.B., Flynn, T.C., Kahrs, R., and Krause, G. Effect of dietary egg on human serum cholesterol and triglycerides. Am J Clin Nutr 1979;32(5):1051–57.
22. Vorster, H.H., Benade, A.J., Barnard, H.C., Locke, M.M., Silvis, N., Venter, C.S., Smuts, C.M., Engelbrecht, G.P., and Marais, M.P. Egg intake does not change plasma lipoprotein and coagulation profiles. Am J Clin Nutr 1992;55(2):400–410.
23. Vorster, H.H., Venter, C.S., Silvis, N., Huisman, H.W., van Ryssen, J.C., Ubbink, J.B., Kotze, J.P., and Walker, A.R. Influence of a habitual high egg intake on serum lipid levels in a rural coloured population. S Afr Med J 1988;74(11):5549.
24. Vorster, H.H., Silvis, N., Venter, C.S., van Ryssen, J.J., Huisman, H., van Eeden, T.S., and Walker, A.R. Serum cholesterol, lipoproteins, and plasma coagulation factors in South Africa blacks on a high-egg but low-fat intake. Am J Clin Nutr 1987;46(1):52–57.
25. Beynen, A.C., and Katan, M.B. Effect of egg yolk feeding on the concentration and composition of serum lipoproteins in man. Atherosclerosis 1985;54(2):157–66.
26. Flynn, M.A., Nolph, G.B., Osio, Y., Sun, G.Y., Lanning, B., Krause, G., and Dally, J.C. Serum lipids and eggs. J Am Diet Assoc 1986;86(11):1541–48.
27. Katan, M.B., Beynen, A.C., de Vries, J.H., and Nobels, A. Existence of cinsistent hypo- and hyperresponder to dietary cholesterol in man. Am J Epidemiol 1986;123(2):221–34.
28. Jacotot, B., Alberich, S., and Motta, C. Effect of dietary monounsaturated fats on HDL fluidity

and composition. In Molecular Biology of Atherosclerosis, Halpern, M.J., ed. London: John Libbey, 1992, pp. 161–64.

29. Buzzard, I.C., Roberts, M.R., Driscol, D.L., and Bowering, J. Effect of dietary eggs and ascorbic acid on plasma lipid and lipoproein cholesterol levels in healthy young men. Am J Clin Nutr 1982;36(1):94–105.
30. Jiang, Z., and Sim, J.S. Effects of dietary n-3 fatty acid-enriched chicken eggs on plasma and tissue cholesterol and fatty acid composition of rats. Lipids 1992;27(4):279–84.
31. Beynen, A.C., and Meijer, G.W. Hyporesponders and hyperresponders to dietary cholesterol. In Molecular Biology of Atherosclerosis, Halpern, M.J., ed. London: John Libbey, 1992, pp. 459–64.
32. Kovanen, P.T., Brown, M.S., Basu, S.K., Bilheimer, D.W., and Goldstein, J.L. Saturation and suppression of hepatic lipoprotein receptors: a mechanism for the hypercholesterolemia of cholesterol-fed rabbits. Proc Natl Acad Sci USA 1981;78(3):1396–1400.
33. Fielding, C.J., Castro, G.R., Donner, C., Fielding, P.E., and Reaven, G.M. Distribution of apolipoprotein E in the plasma of insulin-dependent and noninsulin-dependent diabetics and its relation to cholesterol net transport. J Lipid Res 1986;27(10):1052–61.
34. Venkatesan, S., Imrie, H., Read, S., and Halliday, D. Apo C subclasses from non-insulin-dependent diabetic patients—a quantitative comparison with control subjects. Biochem Soc Trans 1995;23(2):278S.
35. Dawber, T.R., Nickerson, R.J., Brand, F.N., and Pool, J. Eggs, serum cholesterol, and coronary heart disease. Am J Clin Nutr 1982;36(4):617–25.
36. Cliff, W.J. Experiments on animal and human populations. Coronaries Cholesterol. London: Chapman and Hall, 1989, pp. 55–74.
37. Schoefl, G.I. Coronary atherosclerosis: alternative theories of pathogenesis. Coronaries Cholesterol. London: Chapman and Hall: 1989, pp. 26–40.
38. Hansson, G.K., Holm, J., and Jonasson, L. Detection of activated T lymphocytes in the human atherosclerotic plaque. Am J Pathol 1989;135(1):169–75.
39. Frostegard, J., Ulfgren, A.K., Nyberg, P., Hedin, U., Swedenborg, J., Andersson, U., and Hansson, G.K. Cytokine expression in advanced human atherosclerotic plaques: dominance of pro-inflammatory (Th1) and macrophage-stimulating cytokines. Atherosclerosis 1999;145(1):33–43.

11

Eggs and Saturated Fats: Role in Atherosclerosis as Shown by Animal Models

Thomas A. Wilson
and Robert J. Nicolosi

Introduction

Many different animal models have been used to study the effects of dietary saturated fat on lipoprotein concentrations and the development of atherosclerosis. Although, in general, the animal data support observations in humans, they should be interpreted cautiously because (1) certain animal species have lipoprotein profiles during the normal and hypercholesterolemic states that are dissimilar to those of humans, (2) many studies used either no dietary cholesterol or pharmacologic doses, which can significantly influence the size of the fatty acid effect, (3) some diet treatments used variable energy densities, (4) more than one dietary component was varied in a study, and (5) the saturated vegetable oil or fat was substituted for an unsaturated vegetable oil or fat instead of a neutral control.

Animal data for the effects of individual fatty acids on plasma LDL-C concentrations and metabolism and, thus, the development of atherosclerosis are sparse. The evidence suggests that caproic acid (6:0), caprylic acid (8:0), and capric acid (10:0) are neutral with respect to their LDL-C–raising properties and their ability to modulate LDL metabolism. Lauric acid (12:0), myristic acid (14:0), and palmitic acid (16:0) are approximately equivalent in their LDL-C–raising potential by reducing hepatic LDL receptor activity and increasing the LDL-C production rate, apparently via modulation of sterol O-acyltransferase activity. Stearic acid (18:0) appears to be neutral in its LDL-C–raising potential and how it affects LDL metabolism.

For many years, diet-induced hypercholesterolemia as a result of consumption of saturated fat and/or cholesterol feeding was considered an equivalent risk factor for cardiovascular disease. Although in the last several years more emphasis has been given to saturated fat consumption as a result of the greater incremental increase in plasma cholesterol, there are many who continue to argue that dietary cholesterol has an independent effect on atherosclerosis. The epidemiological studies of Stamler and Shekelle[1] and Shekelle and Stamler[2] have often been used to suggest that dietary cholesterol increases the risk for atherosclerosis beyond its plasma LDL-C–raising effects, though to this day the mechanism remains unknown. Although these studies are epidemiological in nature, they are often overinterpreted.

Numerous recent studies have described the effects of saturated fat and individual saturated fatty acids on plasma total and lipoprotein cholesterol concentrations in animal models (for review, see Spady et al.[3]). In contrast, the few recent experimental animal studies that examined the effects of saturated fat on atherosclerosis are not readily available, and virtually no data exists on the influences of individual fatty acids on the atherogenic process. However, one review article summarized several studies conducted nearly four decades ago to test whether different fatty acids added to a cholesterol-enriched diet influenced the incidence and extent of atherosclerosis in hypercholesterolemic rabbits.[4]

While animal studies have shown a clear relationship between saturated fat consumption and atherosclerosis, the association of cholesterol consumption alone with atherosclerosis is less clear because many studies included saturated fat along with the dietary cholesterol and/or fed pharmacological doses of dietary cholesterol.

Steps in the Development of Atherosclerosis

The role of hypercholesterolemia in the development of atherosclerosis as described in the following section represents a synthesis of information derived from the reviews by Ross,[5] Steinberg et al.,[6] and Nicolosi and Stucchi.[7] Elevated serum cholesterol levels associated with the uptake by arteries of atherogenic lipoproteins such as LDL, very low-density lipoprotein (VLDL) remnants, and /or β-VLDL appear to be a necessary prerequisite for initiating atherogenesis (Fig. 11.1). The enhanced uptake of these atherogenic lipoproteins may be associated with nonspecific endothelial dysfunction or with endothelial injury resulting from risk factors such as hypertension, smoking, or diabetes. If endothelial dysfunction exists, once these lipoproteins move into the subintimal space, their residence time may be extended by their interaction with proteoglycan substances that make up the connective tissue matrix of the blood vessel wall and bind avidly to apo B–containing lipoproteins such as LDL and VLDL remnants. This increase in the residence time of these lipoproteins provides a greater opportunity for oxidative modification of LDL. Oxidative LDL acts as a chemoattractant, causing more monocytes to adhere to and penetrate the endothelium. In the presence of endothelial dysfunction, there is increased adhesion of monocytes to the endothelial and movement into the subendothelial space, where they are converted to macrophages. Macrophages, having receptors for modified LDL, can take up more of the modified LDL, forming many intracellular cholesterol ester–laden lipid droplets, ultimately resulting in conversion of the macrophage into a foam cell. The foam cells, engorged with oxidized lipid and apoproteins, may lyse, releasing their content into the extracellular space. This oxidized material is cytotoxic and causes further endothelial injury.

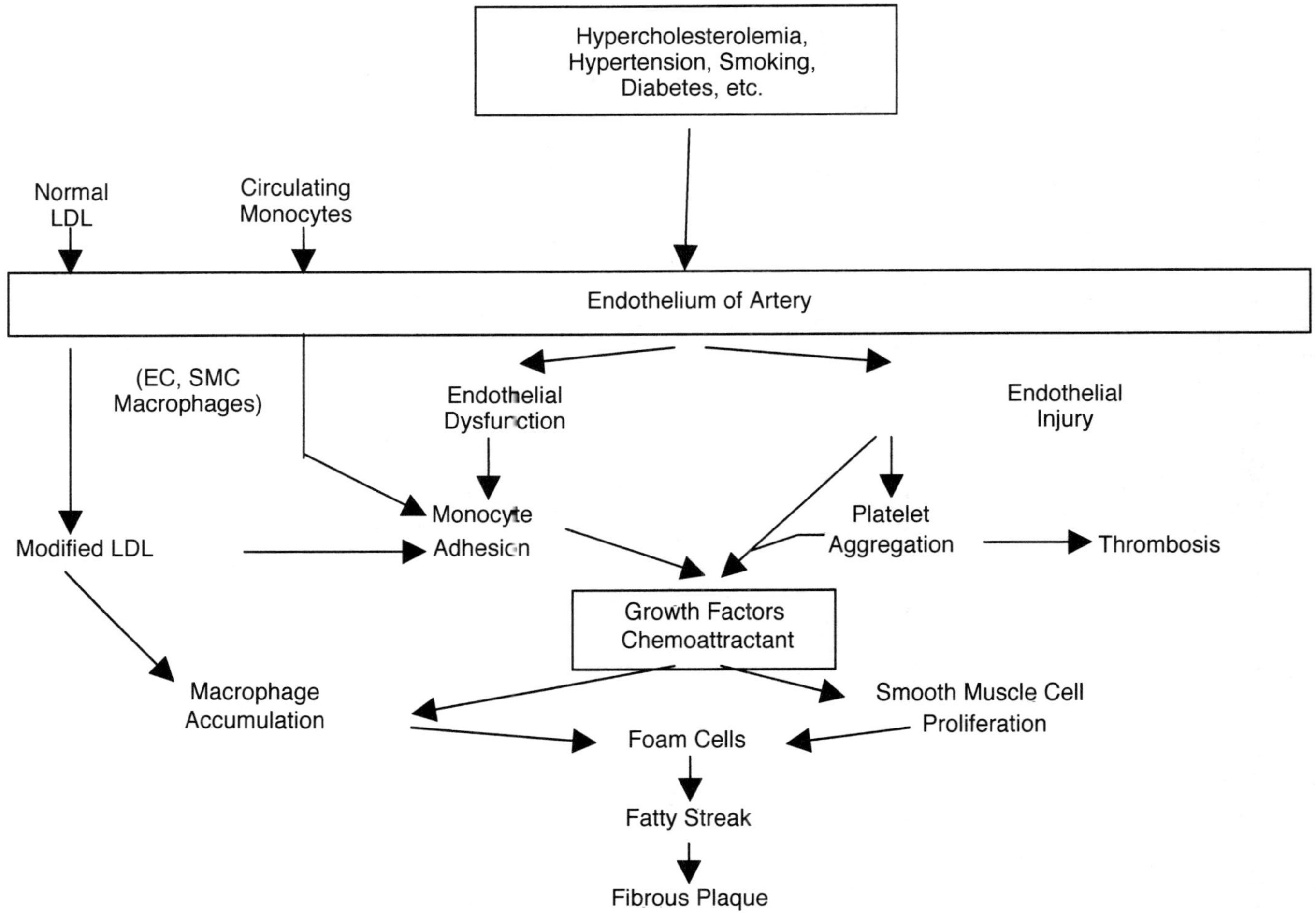

Figure 11.1. Steps in atherosclerosis. LDL = low-density lipoprotein, EC = endothelial cells, and SMC = smooth muscle cells.

Studies of Atherosclerosis in Nonhuman Primates

Nonhuman primates represent an ideal animal model for human atherosclerosis. They develop arterial lesions, which resemble those seen in human beings, and often respond to lipidemic stimulus with the production of lipoproteins resembling those seen in humans. The disadvantages are that nonhuman primates are expensive to purchase and maintain and they are often difficult to handle. Nevertheless, there has been considerable activity in this area of research. The extent of the research effort is a function of consistent availability, and there are now some locally based breeding colonies that assure a reliable, steady supply and that allow for testing of genetic characteristics through selective breeding.

Cebus Monkeys (Cebus albifrons)

Wissler et al.[8] fed cebus monkeys diets containing 0.5 percent cholesterol and 25 percent butterfat, coconut oil, or corn oil. Aortas from all the coconut oil–fed monkeys contained lesions compared with a 75 percent and 0 percent incidence for the butterfat– and corn oil–fed monkeys, respectively.

Rhesus Monkeys (Macaca mulatta)

Almost a half-century ago, Mann and Andrus[9] found that when adult rhesus monkeys were fed a diet high in fat and cholesterol for almost 4 years, they exhibited extensive atherosclerosis of the aorta and all its major branches. The diet was based on dried egg yolk (45 percent) plus 5 percent added cholesterol (providing 6.5 g cholesterol per 100 g diet) and 10 percent corn oil as fat. After 10 months of feeding, serum cholesterol had risen to 1200 mg/dl (31 mM/l) and remained elevated for the duration of the study. The serum ß-lipoproteins (S_f 12-20) were also grossly elevated. The vascular lesions were similar to those seen in human atherosclerosis. In a study with monkeys fed high concentrations of dietary cholesterol (2 percent) and butter, peanut oil, or corn oil (25 percent), less atherosclerosis was found in the monkeys fed corn oil.[10]

Cynomolgus Monkeys (Macaca fascicularis)

The cynomolgus monkey exhibits naturally occurring atherosclerotic lesions.[11] These lesions are present in the aortic arch as well as in the thoracic and abdominal aorta. Diet-induced atherosclerosis in this species was observed by Armstrong,[12] Kramsch and Hollander,[13] and Malinow et al.[14] among others. Wagner et al.[15] found that compared with rhesus monkeys, aortic lesions in cynomolgus monkeys show greater intimal thickening, more extracellular lipid, a greater fibrogenic response, and higher mineral content. Bond et al.[16] also observed myocardial infarctions in cynomolgus monkeys fed a diet containing 25 percent lard and 0.5 percent cholesterol.

African Green (Vervet) Monkeys (Circopithecus aethrops)

The aortic lesions and lipoprotein changes elicited by diet in the African green monkey model resemble those seen in man.[17–19] There is an expanding literature regarding diet and atherosclerosis in the vervet. Much of the data regarding effects of dietary fat on cholesterolemia and atherosclerosis have been accumulated by Rudel and his coworkers.[20–23] They fed vervet monkeys an atherogenic diet (0.8 mg/kcal cholesterol and 40 cal percent as saturated fat) for 11 weeks and then divided them into groups of roughly equal plasma cholesterol and saturated, monounsaturated, or polyunsaturated fat (35 cal percent). There were two phases to the study, one in which monkeys were fed fat mixtures and the other in which they were fed individual fats. Total plasma cholesterol levels were maintained on the saturated fat and fell when the monkeys were fed either mono- or polyunsaturated fat. The relative percentages of LDL- and HDL-cholesterol (high-density lipoprotein–cholesterol) were generally the same on either the mono- or polyunsaturated fat diets with LDL-/HDL-cholesterol ratios between 2.4 and 3.96. In monkeys fed the mixture providing polyunsaturated fat, the LDL/HDL ratio rose to 3.23 (suggesting a drop in HDL-cholesterol levels), whereas in monkeys fed the oleic acid–rich safflower oil it fell to 1.32 (suggesting a fall in the percentage of LDL and a substantial rise in percentage of HDL).[20] Another experiment[21] showed that fish oil, fed for 2.5–3 years, led to lower plasma cholesterol levels than did lard, 231 ± 37 mg/dl (5.97 ± 0.96 mM/l) compared with 360 ± 44 mg/dl (9.31 ± 1.14 mM/l). Aortic atherosclerosis was significantly less severe in the monkeys given fish oil. Subsequent studies showed that feeding polyunsaturated fat from an early age reduced risk for coronary artery atherosclerosis.[22,23]

A study using African green monkeys also supports the atherogenicity of saturated fat.[24] From birth to the age of 5 years, monkeys were fed diets containing 40 percent of energy as fat as either lard (saturated fat) or safflower oil (polyunsaturated fat) with 191 ng cholesterol/J (0.8 mg/kcal). The animals fed the polyunsaturated fat had coronary intimal lesions one-fourth the size of the lesions in animals fed the saturated fat. In addition, the abdominal aorta of the group fed saturated fat contained more sterol clefts and free cholesterol, suggesting more complicated lesions. A similar study in African green monkeys fed 40 percent of energy as fat with 22 percent of energy from the n-3 polyunsaturated fat menhaden oil or from the saturated fat lard with 191 ng cholesterol/J (0.8 mg/kcal) confirmed the atherogenicity of saturated fat.[25] Monkeys fed the diet containing saturated fat for up to 36 months had significantly more coronary artery disease (CAD) and more atherosclerosis in the thoracic aorta and common carotid arteries than did monkeys fed the polyunsaturated fat.

Baboons (Papio ursinus)

There is considerable literature about the effects of diet on blood cholesterol and lipoprotein metabolism in baboons; however, there is relatively little information concerning diet and atherosclerosis development. Gillman and Gilbert[26] published a study of 59 female and 26 male baboons (*Papio ursinus*) aged between 3 and 15 years subsisting on a diet low in cholesterol. From their study they concluded (1) a one to one relationship does not exist between level of dietary fat and serum lipids or between serum lipids and atherosclerosis, (2) accumulation of aortic fat is not necessarily dependent on blood lipids but appears to be secondary to alterations in the aortic tissue that favor binding fat and calcium, and (3) the functional and structural integrity of the intima and media are determined not only by their intrinsic properties but also by factors arising beyond the vascular tree.

McGill, Jr., et al.[27] examined the arteries of 163 free-ranging Kenyan baboons and found that about 75 percent of the adults exhibited some degree of fatty streaking in the aorta. The amount of streaking increased with age. Strong and McGill, Jr.,[28] fed baboons high-cholesterol diets for 2 years. Serum cholesterol increased moderately, and there were some fatty streaks but no advanced lesions. A 4-year experiment in which a diet high in fat and cholesterol was fed[29] led to moderate cholesterolemia, but on necropsy, the principal lesion was still only a fatty streak. Cholesterol-fed baboons exhibited a positive relationship between aortic fatty streaks and elevated serum levels of LDL- and VLDL-cholesterol. There was also a negative relationship between HDL-cholesterol levels and aortic fatty streaks.[30]

In many of these studies, fat was fed along with high concentrations of cholesterol, making it difficult to identify relative contributions of the different dietary fats to atherogenesis. However, in one study in which squirrel and cebus monkeys were fed the saturated fat coconut oil but no dietary cholesterol, elevated plasma cholesterol concentrations were associated in squirrel monkeys with significant atherosclerosis compared with monkeys fed corn oil.[31] Similarly, cynomolgus monkeys fed 41 percent of energy as fat (butter, olive and corn oil) with 0.1 percent cholesterol had significantly more atherosclerosis than did monkeys fed a diet in which butter was replaced with peanut oil.[32]

The foregoing studies suggest that primate models of atherosclerosis are variable and can be influenced by diet and stress. A major aim of human studies is to effect regression of pre-established lesions. Regression of atherosclerosis in primates has been reviewed by Stary[33] and Malinow.[34] Reversion of primates from an atherogenic diet to one low in fat and cholesterol will lead to diminution of lesion severity in rhesus and cynomolgus monkeys. Wagner et al.[35] fed rhesus monkeys an atherogenic diet for 19 months. Twelve animals were necropsied at 19 months to provide baseline data. The remaining 36 monkeys were fed diets designed to maintain their plasma cholesterol levels at about 200 or 300 mg/dl for an additional 48 months. More cholesterol was lost from arteries of monkeys maintained at 200 mg/dl than those kept at 300 mg/dl. Eggen et al.[36] have shown that pre-established lesions in rhesus monkeys can regress even when fed a diet free of cholesterol but high in saturated fat for 30 or 52 weeks. Vesselinovitch et al.[37] have demonstrated that rhesus monkeys fed a prudent diet exhibit about 70 percent fewer aortic lesions than those fed an atherogenic diet for 14 months and 77 percent fewer lesions than monkeys fed the same diet for 48 months. The primate model is useful for the study of both progression and regression of atherosclerosis, and it is closer to humans than the other available models.

Studies of Atherosclerosis in Rodents

In rodent studies, the effect of feeding saturated fat is often evaluated in animals fed high concentrations of cholesterol, which makes identifying the specific fat effects impossible.

Hamsters

In one study, hamsters were fed coconut oil along with high concentrations of dietary cholesterol (3 percent), which prevented assessing different dietary fat effects on atherosclerosis.[38] However, in other studies, this same saturated fat was shown to produce early atherosclerosis at more typical concentrations of dietary cholesterol.[39,40] Recently in a study conducted in our laboratory,[41] golden Syrian hamsters were fed diets containing various levels of dietary coconut oil (saturated fat) or cholesterol and 10 percent cocoa butter (neutral fat) for 10 weeks. When the data were compared based on similar plasma LDL-C, the hamsters fed the cholesterol-containing diets had significantly less early atherosclerosis compared with the animals fed the coconut oil-containing diets, at lower plasma LDL-C levels (<1.3 mmol/l). However, at higher plasma LDL-C (>1.9 mmol/l), the hamsters fed the cholesterol-containing diets had early atherosclerosis significantly more often than hamsters fed the coconut oil–containing diets.

In a recent study,[42] hamsters were fed a diet containing 20 percent total fat and 0.12 percent cholesterol where the different test diets contained either 8:0, 14:0, *cis*-18:1, or *trans*-18:1 at approximately 50 percent of the total fat. While plasma LDL-C concentrations were significantly higher in the 14:0 diet only, formation of early atherosclerotic lesions was greater in both the 14:0 and 8:0 diets compared with the other diets.

Rabbits

For rabbits with comparable serum cholesterol concentrations, a diet containing cholesterol and methyl stearate was more atherogenic than diets containing methyl oleate or methyl linoleate.[43] A study on the effects of naturally occurring fats on pre-established atheroma in rabbits fed 2 percent cholesterol and either 5 percent corn oil or coconut oil found that corn oil retarded the progression of lesions relative to coconut oil.[44] In another series of investigations examining the effects of fat saturation on atherosclerosis in rabbits with comparable serum cholesterol concentrations, palm oil feeding resulted in more atherogenesis than did cocoa butter feeding, but both produced more severe lesions than did corn oil treatment.[45] In a similar experiment with rabbits, palm oil was found to be as atherogenic as coconut oil, and cocoa butter was more atherogenic than corn oil but less than coconut and palm oils.[46] This raised the question of whether 12:0, 14:0, 16:0, and 18:0 affect atherogenicity differently.

To address this question, for several weeks rabbits were fed corn oil or corn oil in which the triacylglycerol structure was interesterified with 12:0, 14:0, 16:0, and 18:0, and atherogenesis was then evaluated. A measure of the atherogenic index revealed that 12:0-, 14:0-, and 16:0-enriched diets produced more atherosclerosis than did the 18:0-enriched diet, but that all were higher than the index for the control corn oil diet.[47] In swine fed butter or two different concentrations of corn oil for 12 weeks, the reductions in serum cholesterol concentrations for both corn oil treatment groups relative to butter were accompanied by rather striking decreases in atherogenesis.[48]

Apo E–Knockout Mice

Apolipoprotein E3-Leiden (APO) transgenic mice develop hyperlipidemia and are highly susceptible to diet-induced atherosclerosis. The progression and histopathology of lesions in this animal model show similar features to those observed in humans and other species, including fatty streaks, necrotic cores, and fibrous caps.[49–51]

Calleja et al.[52] investigated the effect of palm, coconut, olive, and sunflower oils (10 percent wt/wt) without the addition of cholesterol for 10 weeks on the development of atherosclerosis in apo E–knockout mice. None of the diets induced changes in plasma cholesterol concentrations, whereas plasma triglycerides were uniformly reduced in all diet groups. Some diets caused significant reductions in the size of atherosclerotic lesions in males and others in females; males responded most to sunflower oil and females to palm and olive oils.

In another study,[53] apo E-knockout mice were fed a diet containing 15 percent cocoa butter, 0.5 percent cholate, and 1 percent cholesterol for 12 months. After 12 months on the diet, lesions in the aortic arch showed calcification and lesions with a fibrous cap were observed at both the right and left carotid artery bifurcations. Moreover, 5 of 12 mice showed calcifications in their coronary arteries. Groot et al.[54] investigated APOE*3 Leiden mice fed a high–saturated fat/high-cholesterol/0.5 percent cholate diet for 6 months. They observed 5 to 10 times greater lesion areas in transgenic mice compared with nontransgenic mice.

Eggs and Cholesterol Consumption and Atherosclerosis in Animal Models

In the majority of animal studies that examined the influence of eggs/egg yolk consumption on plasma cholesterol levels and the development of atherosclerosis, eggs were used for the single purpose of being a dietary source of cholesterol to produce a hypercholesterolemic state in the animal model. However, a few studies did examine the direct effect of feeding eggs/egg yolk on plasma cholesterol levels.

In a study conducted by Srilatha et al.,[55] healthy, nonobese, young rabbits developed hypercholesterolemia following daily intake of fresh egg yolk for 8 weeks. On a quantitative basis, this diet had a profound effect on serum cholesterol level, which rose to 15 or 30 times the baseline value depending on whether the test group consumed the yolk content of one or two eggs during the study. In another study,[56] the feeding of powdered versus fresh egg yolks to young male chickens up to 30 and 43 weeks of age, respectively, produced approximately the same increase in plasma cholesterol, liver fat, and liver cholesterol when compared with the feeding of a soybean-based cholesterol-free diet. Also, aortic atherosclerosis, however, was found to be more severe in a group of birds fed fresh egg yolks than in those fed powdered egg or the cholesterol-free diet.[56]

However, when consuming eggs or egg yolks, dietary cholesterol is not the only nutrient that is consumed. Other possible cholesterol-lowering nutrients, such as lecithin, are found in sufficient quantities in eggs. O'Brien and Corrigan[57] compared the influence on plasma and tissue lipids of dietary soybean and egg lecithins, which have contrasting fatty acid compositions, in hypercholesterolemic guinea pigs. Among the most noteworthy observations were the 49 percent decrease in total plasma cholesterol of animals fed 7.5 percent soybean lecithin without decreasing HDL-C and the 177 percent increase in plasma HDL-C of the animals fed 7.5 percent egg lecithin without a significant increase in total cholesterol compared with control-fed animals.[57]

Conclusion

There are substantial data related to the hypercholesterolemic properties of animal fat and vegetable oils that contain high amounts of saturated fatty acids. Early studies conducted mostly in rabbits but also pigs and monkeys indicate that diet-induced hypercholesterolemia is associated with atherosclerosis. These studies suggest that, in general, the atherogenicity is comparable for animal fat and vegetable oils enriched in 12:0, 14:0, and 16:0, and the atherogenicity of these is greater than that of fats enriched in 18:0. The data relating specific fatty acids to atherosclerosis are sparse, and although the relative effects of 12:0, 14:0, and 16:0 appear to be similar collectively (and probably individually), they are more atherogenic than 18:0. Additional studies are needed to clarify the cholesterolemic and atherogenic effects of the individual saturated fatty acids.

While consumption of eggs, particularly egg yolks, has become a concern for most people because of their dietary cholesterol, there are many other nutrients that may have other beneficial health effects for humans. Most recent is the development of chicken eggs that have been naturally incorporated with omega-3 polyunsaturated fatty acids through the chickens' diet.

Acknowledgment

The authors wish to thanks Susan Ralls for manuscript preparation.

References

1. Stamler, J., and Shekelle, R. Dietary cholesterol and human coronary heart disease. Arch Pathol Lab Med 1988;112:1032.
2. Shekelle, R. and Stamler, J. Dietary cholesterol and ischaemic heart disease. Lancet 1989;1:1177.

3. Spady, D.K., Woollett, L.A., and Dietschy, J.M. Regulation of plasma LDL-cholesterol levels by dietary cholesterol and fatty acids. Annu Rev Nutr 1993;13:355.
4. Kritchevsky, D. Role of cholesterol vehicle in experimental atherosclerosis. Am J Clin Nutr 1970;23:1105.
5. Ross, R. The pathogenesis of atherosclerosis—an update. N Engl J Med 1986;314:488.
6. Steinberg, D., Parthasarathy, S., Carew, T.E., Khoo, J.C., and Witztum, J.L. Modifications of low-density lipoprotein that increase its atherogenicity. N Engl J Med 1989;320:915.
7. Nicolosi, R.J., and Stucchi, A.F. n-3 Fatty acids and atherosclerosis. Curr Opin Lipidol 1990;1:442.
8. Wissler, R.W., Frazier, L.E., Hughes, R.H., and Rasmussen, R.A. Atherogenesis in the cebus monkey I. A comparison of three food fats under controlled dietary conditions. Arch Pathol 1962;74:312.
9. Mann, G.V., and Andrus, S.B. Xanthomatosis and atherosclerosis produced by diet in an adult rhesus monkey. J Lab Clin Med 1956;48:533.
10. Vesselinovitch, D., Getz, G.S., Hughes, R.H., and Wissler, R.W. Atherosclerosis in the rhesus monkey fed three food fats. Atherosclerosis 1974;20:303.
11. Pathap, K. Spontaneous aortic lesions in wild adult Malaysian long-tailed monkeys (*Macaca irus*). J Pathol 1973;110:135.
12. Armstrong, M.L. Atherosclerosis in rhesus and cynomolgus monkeys. Primates Med 1976;9:16.
13. Kramsch, D., and Hollander, W. Occlusive atherosclerotic disease of the coronary arteries in monkeys (*Macaca irus*) induced by diet. Exp Mol Pathol 1968;9:1.
14. Malinow, M.R., et al. A model for therapeutic interventions on established coronary atherosclerosis in a non-human primate. Adv Exp Med Biol 1976;67:3.
15. Wagner, W.D., St. Clair, R.W., and Clarkson, T.B. Angiochemical and tissue cholesterol changes in *Macaca fascicularis* fed an atherogenic diet for three years. Exp Mol Pathol 1978;28:140.
16. Bond, M.G., et al. Myocardial infarction in a large colony of non-human primates with coronary artery atherosclerosis. Am J Pathol 1980;101:675.
17. Clarkson, T.B. Arteriosclerosis of African green and stump-tailed macaque monkeys. In Atherosclerosis III, Achettler, G., and Weizel, A., eds. New York: Springer-Verlag, 1974, p. 291.
18. Bullock, B.C., et al. Comparative primate atherosclerosis I. Tissue cholesterol concentrations and pathologic anatomy. Exp Mol Pathol 1975;22:151.
19. Wagner, W.D., and Clarkson, T.B. Comparative primate atherosclerosis II. A biochemical study of lipids, calcium and collagen in atherosclerotic arteries. Exp Mol Pathol 1975;23:96.
20. Rudel, L.L., Haines, J.L., and Sawyer, J.K. Effects on plasma lipoproteins of monounsaturated, saturated, and polyunsaturated fatty acids in the diet of African green monkeys. J Lipid Res 1990;31:1873.
21. Parker, J.S., et al. Effects of dietary fish oil on coronary artery and aortic atherosclerosis in African green monkeys. Arteriosclerosis 1990;10;1102.
22. Wolfe, M.S., et al. Childhood consumption of dietary polyunsaturated fat lowers risk for coronary artery atherosclerosis in African green monkeys. Arterioscler Thromb 1993;13:863.
23. Rudel, L.L., Parks, J.S., and Sawyer, J.K. Compared with dietary monounsaturated and saturated fat, polyunsaturated fat protects African green monkeys from coronary artery atherosclerosis. Arterioscler Thromb Vasc Biol 1995;15:2101.
24. Wolfe, M.S., et al. Dietary polyunsaturated fat decreases coronary artery atherosclerosis in a pediatric-aged population of African green monkeys. Arterioscler Thromb 1994;14:587.

25. Parks, J.S., et al. Effect of dietary fish oil on coronary artery and aortic atherosclerosis in African green monkeys, Atherosclerosis 1990;10:1102.
26. Gillman, J., and Gilbert, C. Atheroslerosis in the baboon (*Papio ursinus*). Its pathogenesis and etiology. Exp Med Surg 1957;15:181.
27. McGill, H.C., Jr., et al. Arterial lesions in the Kenya baboon. Circ Res 1960;8:670.
28. Strong, J.P., and McGill, H.C., Jr. Diet and experimental atherosclerosis in baboons. Am J Pathol 1967;50:669.
29. Strong, J.P., Eggen, D.A., and Jirge, S.K. Atherosclerotic lesions produced in baboons by feeding an atherogenic diet for four years. Exp Mol Pathol 1976;24:320.
30. McGill, H.C., Jr., et al. Relationship of lipoprotein cholesterol concentrations to experimental atherosclerosis in baboons. Arteriosclerosis 1981;1:3.
31. Nicolosi, R.J., et al. Diet and lipoprotein influence on primate atherosclerosis. Proc Soc Exp Biol Med 1977;156:1.
32. Anderson, L.M., Hayes, K.C., and Nicolosi, R.J. Peanut oil reduces diet-induced atherosclerosis in cynomolgus monkeys. Arteriosclerosis 1986;6:465.
33. Stary, H.C. Regression of atherosclerosis in primates. Virchows Arch Pathol Anat Histol 1979;383:117.
34. Malinow, M.R. Atherosclerosis. Regression in non-human primates. Circ Res 1980;46:311.
35. Wagner, W.D., et al. A study of atherosclerosis regression in *Macaca mulatta*. Am J Pathol 1980;100:633.
36. Eggen, D.A., et al. Regression of experimental atherosclerotic lesions in rhesus monkeys consuming a high saturated fat diet. Arteriosclerosis 1987;7:125.
37. Vesselinovitch, D., Wissler, R.W., and Schaffner, T.J. Quantitation of lesions during progression and regression of atherosclerosis in rhesus monkeys. In Nutrition and Heart Disease, Naito, H.K., ed. New York: SP Medical and Scientific Books, 1982, p. 121.
38. Nistor, A., et al. The hyperlipidemic hamster as a model of experimental atherosclerosis. Atherosclerosis 1987;68:159.
39. Kowala, M.C., et al. Doxazosin and cholestyramine similarly decrease fatty streak formation in the aortic arch of hyperlipidemic hamsters. Atherosclerosis 1991;91:35.
40. Foxall, T.L., et al. Dose-response effects of doxazosin on plasma lipids and aortic fatty streak formation in the hypercholesterolemic hamster model. Am J Pathol 1992;140:1357.
41. Winchester, L., et al. Does saturated fat have a greater influence on the development of atherosclerosis than cholesterol. J Am Coll Nutr 1999;18:553.
42. Nicolosi, R.J., et al. Effects of specific fatty acids (8:0, 14:0, *cis*-18:1, *trans*-18:1) on plasma lipoproteins, early atherogenic potential, and LDL oxidative properties in the hamster. J Lipid Res 1998;39:1972.
43. Kritchevsky, D., et al. Effect of cholesterol vehicle in experimental atherosclerosis. Am J Physiol 1954;178:30.
44. Kritchevsky, D., and Tepper, S.A. Effect of coconut oil on pre-established atheroma in rabbits. Naturwissenschaften 1964;51:313.
45. Kritchevsky, D., and Tepper, S.A. Cholesterol vehicle in experimental atherosclerosis. VII. Influence of naturally occurring saturated fatty acids. Med Pharmacol Exp 1965;12:315.
46. Kritchevsky, D. Cholesterol vehicle in experimental atherosclerosis. Acad Med N J Bull 1966;12:157.
47. Kritchevsky, D., and Tepper, S.A. Cholesterol vehicle in experimental atherosclerosis. X. Influence of specific occurring saturated fatty acids. Exp Mol Pathol 1967:394.

48. Kim, D.N., et al. Hypo-atherogenic effect of dietary corn oil exceeds hypo-cholesterolemic effect in swine. Atherosclerosis 1984;52:101.
49. Zhang, S.H., et al. Spontaneous hypercholesterolemia and arterial lesion in mice lacking apolipoprotein E. Science 1992;258:468.
50. Nakashima, Y., et al. Apo E-deficient mice develop lesions of all phases of atherosclerosis throughout the atrial tree. Arterioscler Thromb 1994;14:133.
51. Reddick, R.L., Zhang, S.H., and Maeda, N. Atherosclerosis in mice lacking apo E. Evaluation of lesional development and progression. Arterioscler Thromb 1994;14:141.
52. Calleja, L., et al. Low-cholesterol and high-fat diets reduce atherosclerotic lesion development in apo E-knockout mice. Arterioscler Thromb Vasc Biol 1999;19:2368.
53. Lutgens, E., et al. Atherosclerosis in APOE*3-Leiden transgenic mice. From proliferative to atheromatous stage. Circulation 1999;99:276.
54. Groot, P.H., et al. Quantitative assessment of aortic atherosclerosis in APOE*3 Leiden transgenic mice and its relationship to serum cholesterol exposure. Arterioscler Thromb Vasc Biol 1996;16:926.
55. Srilatha, B., Adaikan, P.G., and Aulkumaran, S. Effects of feeding egg yolk on the serum lipid levels in rabbits. Methods Find Exp Clin Pharmacol 1997;19:489.
56. Griminger, P., and Fisher, H. The effect of dried and fresh eggs on plasma cholesterol and atherosclerosis in chickens. Poult Sci 1986;65:979.
57. O'Brien, S.C., and Corrigan, S.M. The influence of dietary soybean and egg lecithins on lipid responses in cholesterol-fed guinea pigs. Lipids 1988;23:647.

12

Health Effects of Docosahexanoic Acid (DHA)–Enriched Eggs

Jin Zhang
and Ronald R. Watson

INTRODUCTION

Docosahexanoic acid (DHA, 22:5 n-3), one of the major n-3 long-chain polyunsaturated fatty acids (LCPUFAs), is essential for the growth and functional development of the brain in infants as well as for maintenance of normal brain function in adults. The inclusion of plentiful DHA in the diet improves learning ability, whereas deficiencies of DHA are associated with deficits in learning. DHA is good for the eyes and helpful in recovery from certain visual dysfunctions. The visual acuity of healthy, full-term, formula-fed infants is increased when their formula includes DHA. DHA also has a positive effect on diseases such as heart disease, thrombosis, and atherosclerosis.

Humans obtain DHA primarily from their diets because they are capable of synthesizing only small amounts of DHA.[1] Therefore, researchers have explored a variety of food supplements. This chapter discusses how DHA-enriched eggs promote health. The nutritional manipulation of the diets of laying hens to include sources of n-3 fatty acids (FAs) promotes the deposition of these nutrients into egg yolk.[2] Therefore, DHA-rich eggs may provide an exciting alternative food source for enhancing consumer intake of these healthful FAs.

INTERACTIONS BETWEEN POLYUNSATURATED FATTY ACIDS (PUFAS)

Fat is an essential component of the human diet. The essential fatty acids are the critical components of fat. Essential fatty acids include linoleic acid (LA) and its n-6 derivative, arachidonic acid (AA). More recently, the vital role of α-linolenic acid (α-LNA) and its n-3 derivative, DHA, has been recognized.[1] The active components in both series are the longer-chain acids such as AA and DHA. These are produced by desaturation and elongation or obtained from the diet. A high ratio of LA to α-LNA causes a depletion of the longer-chain n-3 fatty acids (FAs), including DHA, by competing for the enzymes necessary for desaturation and elongation.[3]

Humans originally consumed a diet rich in the n-3 FAs and low in saturated FAs because wild and free-range food animals have much higher contents of n-3 FAs than do present-day commercial livestock. The dietary supply of FAs previously contained a 1:1 ratio of n-6 to n-3 PUFAs.[1] The present ratio in the United States is greater than 10:1, causing a deficiency of the n-3 FAs. An increased intake of LA and an elevated ratio of n-6 to n-3 FA is a major risk factor for Western-type cancers, thrombosis diseases, apoplexy, and allergic hypersensitivity.[1] The World Health Organization is now recommending a ratio of between 3:1 and 4:1 for n-6 to n-3 FAs, an increase of the n-3 FAs portion in the human diet. As we know, dietary α-LNA can be metabolically converted to DHA; however, the enzymes involved in this conversion are common to the pathway for the elongation and desaturation of LA, and competition with n-6 FAs will reduce the amount of α-LNA converted (Fig. 12.1).[3,4]

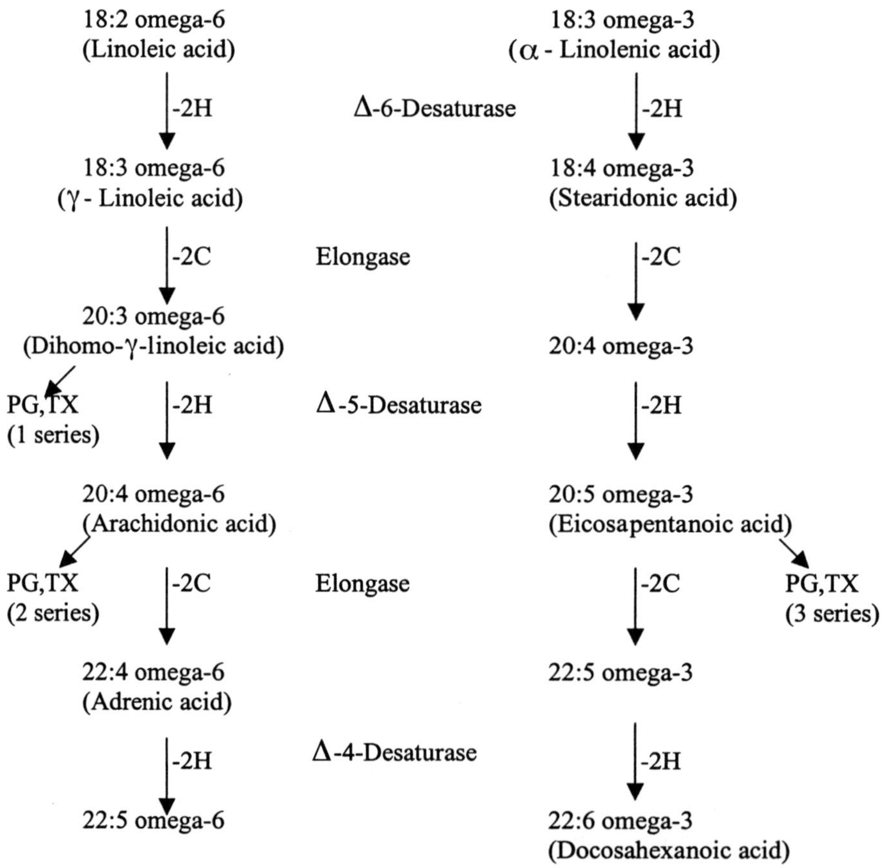

Figure 12.1. Interactions among polyunsaturated fatty acids. Modified from Reference 3.

Food Sources of DHA

DHA is more prevalent in fatty fish (salmon, tuna, and mackerel) than in meat and eggs. DHA is usually present in human milk instead of in infant formula.[1] Eicosapentanoic acid (EPA), another long-chain n-3 fatty acid, also exists in fatty fish. However, fish is not consumed regularly or in large quantities in many Western countries.[5] In the United Kingdom and the United States, daily average intakes of DHA and EPA are extremely small, and a dietary insufficiency of n-3 PUFAs is likely to occur.

Fish oil is currently the primary dietary source of EPA and DHA, which is associated with reduced cardiovascular diseases. However, fish oil consumption is still very limited due to availability and cost.[6,18] Various sources of DHA have been developed for human DHA intake. Poultry meat is often an important source of these n-3 PUFAs in the United States because fishmeal may be added to poultry diets.[5]

Other forms of DHA are now being developed. It is well-known that the composition of the fatty acids in egg yolk can be altered.[5] Eggs enriched with DHA are on the market in several countries. Woobang Science Company, Ltd., is now producing Edison 300TM eggs, containing at least 300 mg DHA per 100 g of egg, in Korea. This company provided a feed supplement for laying hens containing fish oil, flaxseed, and a mixture that stimulates the conversion of n-3 PUFAs to DHA.[6] Experiments were also conducted to investigate the usefulness of a natural golden marine algae (MA) as a poultry ration supplement for the production of shell eggs rich in n-3 FAs.[7] A fermentation production technology for *Schizochytrium* was developed that utilized inexpensive nutrients and achieved high culture densities, short production cycles, and very high concentrations of DHA in the algae. DHA-enriched eggs were produced by feeding dried *Schizochytrium* fermentation products to laying hens (Table 12.1).[8,9] Because eggs can be made into so many products, eggs enriched with DHA by feeding hens a microalgal feed source provide consumers with a wider variety of food sources containing DHA than does fish oil or flaxseed.[10] Research on the DHA enrichment of eggs and their effects on humans as they consumed these eggs and egg products has been conducted in several areas.

Health Benefits of DHA

Nervous System in Infants

The brain is 60 percent structural lipid, which universally uses AA (20:4n-6) and DHA (22:6n-3) for growth, function, and integrity.[11] Experimental evidence in animals has demonstrated that the effect of essential fatty acid deficiency during early brain development is deleterious and permanent. The risk of neurodevelopment disorder is highest in the very low birth weight babies. Babies born with low birth weight or prematurely are most likely to have been born to mothers who were inadequately nourished, and the babies tend to be born with AA and DHA deficits. Because brain development disorders can be permanent, proper provision should be made to protect the AA and DHA status of both term and preterm infants to ensure optimum conditions for the development of membrane-

Table 12.1. Lipid components in DHA-enriched eggs laying hens

Lipids	Market egg	DHA egg
Saturated fatty acids		
C14:0	34	50
C16:0	2,226	2,310
C18:0	784	790
C20:0	10	<10
C22:0	12	<10
Monounsaturated fatty acids		
C14:1	8	<10
C16:1	298	300
C18:1	3,473	3,530
C20:1	28	20
C22:1	3	<10
Polyunsaturated fatty acids		
C18:2 n-6	1,148	1,100
C18:3 n-3	33	150
C20:4 n-6	142	100
C22:6 n-3	37	[a]270
Cholesterol	425	455

Source. Modified from Reference 9.
[a]Significantly different content between market and DHA eggs.

rich systems such as the brain and the nervous and vascular systems. Another evidence of DHA physiological function in nervous tissue membrane is that the concentration of DHA in the membranes of the retina and brain is very high and the deficiency of DHA results in loss of visual acuity in monkeys and human infants.[4]

DHA plays an important role in the maintenance of normal neural functions, a role that n-6 FAs cannot fill. The outgrowth of neurites induced by nerve growth factor is promoted by DHA. Part of the unique function of DHA in the nervous system seems to relate to the synthesis of phospholipids (PLs) for the membranes needed for neurite elongation.[1] During fetal development, DHA can be preferentially transported across the placenta into the fetal circulation to match the requirement of fetal growth, especially in the brain and vascular systems.[12] DHA deficits may lead to deficits in learning ability because DHA is involved in cell signaling. DHA is the predominant structural FA in the brain's gray matter and retinal tissues in humans and other mammals.[1] Infant brain growth requires the formation of large amounts of neural membrane. Synaptic membranes are especially rich in two LCPUFAs: DHA and AA. Potential sources of LCPUFA for supplementation include fish oils and egg lipids. In animal studies dietary shortages of both DHA and its precursor α-LNA have resulted in reduced levels of DHA in the brain and adverse effects on early brain development (e.g., visual deficits in a primate model and altered learning behaviors in a rat model).[13]

Many independent studies indicate that the mental development and visual acuity of infants are positively affected by breast-feeding and that breast-fed infants have higher levels of DHA in the brain tissues and enhanced mental ability later in life when compared with those fed infant formula not containing DHA.[1] A study was done to determine whether DHA supplementation of breast-feeding mothers increases the DHA contents of breast milk and infant plasma PLs. Breast-feeding women were randomly assigned to three DHA-supplementation groups (170–260 mg/d) and a control group.[14] Group 1 (n = 6) consumed an algae-produced high-DHA triacylglycerol; group 2 (n = 6) consumed high-DHA eggs; group 3 (n = 6) consumed a high-DHA, low-EPA marine oil; and group 4 (n = 6) received no supplementation. Correlations between the DHA contents of maternal plasma and breast milk and of milk and infant PLs were significant. Breast milk and maternal and infant PL 22:5n-6 concentrations were lowest in group 2. DHA supplementation increases the plasma and breast milk DHA concentrations of lactating women, resulting in higher PL DHA concentrations in infants. There were significant correlations between the contents of all long-chain (containing >18 carbons) n-3 and n-6 polyunsaturated fatty acids in maternal plasma phospholipids and the contents of these fatty acids in milk. The correlation between maternal plasma phospholipid DHA and milk DHA was particularly strong. Similar, although weaker, correlations were observed between the contents of these fatty acids in milk and those in infant plasma phospholipids.

Since DHA is not available in most infant formulas, supplementing could be an alternative source of DHA. For example, eggs laid from Greek chickens (called Greek eggs) contain more DHA (22:6 n-3) and less LA (18:2 n-6) and LNA (18:3 n-3) than do eggs from hens fed fish meal or flaxseed. Two to 3 g of Greek egg yolk may provide an adequate amount of DHA and AA for a preterm neonate.[15] With proper manipulation of the hens' diets, eggs could be produced with FA composition similar to that of Greek eggs as a source of DHA to supplement infant formula.

Cardio-Protective Effects

The leading cause of death in Western countries is cardiovascular disease.[16] The increase in deaths due to coronary heart disease in these countries has been blamed on the increased consumption of saturated fats. The American Heart Association estimates that 57 million Americans have cardiovascular disease, causing 954,000 deaths annually and costing $259 billion per year. Many billions of dollars are spent annually on developing drugs. Although drugs such as cholestyramine and clolibrate are effective in reducing triglycerides and LDL-cholesterol and increasing HDL-cholesterol, they have significant side effects. Better nutrition with plenty of long-chain n-3 FAs, especially DHA, can produce the same lipid changes and positive effects with no side effects and much less expense.

Epidemiological studies have shown a strong correlation between fish consumption and reduction in sudden death from myocardial infarction. The reduction is approximately 50 percent with 200 mg per day of DHA from fish. DHA is the principal active component in fish for cardiovascular protection.[17] DHA supplements increase the HDL-/LDL-cholesterol ratio and decrease the total cholesterol/HDL ratio, suggesting a decreased risk for coronary artery disease. Even an intake of only 2.9 g of EPA and DHA per month was associated with a 30 percent reduced risk. Blood samples taken after 16 and 22 weeks from fasting subjects showed significant increases in EPA, DHA, and total n-3 PUFAs in subjects consuming enriched eggs compared with controls.[5] Serum triglyceride concentrations in human subjects consuming the n-3 fatty acids EPA plus DHA are consistently reduced, and platelet n-3 fatty acids consistently increased.[4] In addition, the ratio of n-6 to n-3 PUFAs in plasma was significantly reduced from 12.2:1 to 6.5–7.7:1 in subjects consuming enriched eggs compared with controls (Table 12.2). Consumption of only one enriched egg daily can contribute substantially to the recommended daily intake of n-3 PUFAs. Moderate lowering of plasma triglyceride concentrations was observed in human subjects consuming eggs enriched in EPA and DHA from hens fed fish oil. Feeding hens ground flaxseed has produced eggs high in α-LNA. Although less pronounced than for α-LNA, the DHA concentration is also significantly increased in these eggs.[4]

Platelet function and blood coagulation play important roles in coronary artery disease. Flaxseed oil decreased collagen-induced platelet aggregation and thromboxane production.[4] Both platelets from human subjects consuming DHA and human platelets incubated in vitro with DHA exhibited depressed platelet reactivity. Excessive platelet aggregation can lead to arterial thrombosis, while n-3 FAs are associated with reduced platelet aggregations as well as the risk of coronary heart disease. The accumulation of DHA PLs, as observed for modified-egg consumers, provided some added health benefits in addition to its role in neuronal functioning. Additionally, EPA can inhibit the aggregation of blood platelets, an important factor in reducing the incidence of cardiovascular disease. DHA can also fulfill this function through retroconversion to EPA. The intermediate compound in this process is docosapentanoic acid (DPA).[5]

On the other hand, in the pathogenesis of atherosclerosis, vascular smooth muscle cell growth is an important component. These cells have the potential to proliferate and accumulate lipids. Cyclins and cyclin-dependent kinases control progression through the eukaryotic cell cycle and thus the proliferation of cells. DHA and EPA inhibit DNA synthesis through G1 cyclins, cyclin-dependent kinase inhibitor (p27), and stop the progression from the G1 to the S phase. By this mechanism, DHA and EPA inhibit the proliferation of vascular smooth muscle cells.[1]

Conclusion

Eggs are not only widely accepted as cheap and complete nutritional packages but also can now be used to meet a substantial part of the recommended dietary intake of n-3 PUFAs because the ratio of n-6 to n-3 FAs can be properly balanced by ingesting specialized hen eggs. Attempts have been made to produce eggs that are rich in DHA; such eggs have been shown to not raise cholesterol and lower the ratio of n-6 to n-3 (Table 12.1). Upon consumption of DHA-enriched eggs, serum and platelet lipid alterations have been associated with a reduced risk of myocardial infarction and thrombosis. People on a Western diet may also improve their cardiovascular risk factors by consuming DHA-

Table 12.2. Fatty acid composition of lipid in control and modified eggs

	Amount of flax in diet of hen		
Fatty acid	0%	10%	20%
	(% by wt. of total fatty acids)		
16:0	23.3 ± 0.5	22.5 ± 0.3	21.0 ± 0.4
16:1	2.1 ± 0.2	2.4 ± 0.3	3.0 ± 0.3
18:0	7.8 ± 0.1	8.1 ± 0.1	6.3 ± 0.8
18:1	40.8 ± 0.9	39.4 ± 0.6	36.5 ± 1.2
18:2n-6	16.8 ± 1.1	15.2 ± 0.4	16.3 ± 0.5
18:3n-6 (α-LNA)	0.5 ± 0.04	5.5 ± 0.4	10.7 ± 0.4
20:4n-6	2.2 ± 0.16	1.1 ± 0.1	0.9 ± 0.06
20:5n-3 (EPA)	0.1 ± 0.05	0.2 ± 0.05	0.2 ± 0.03
22:4n-6	0.4 ± 0.07	0.3 ± 0.02	0.2 ± 0.04
22:5n-3 (DPA)	0.2 ± 0.05	0.3 ± 0.03	0.4 ± 0.1
22:6n-3 (DHA)	1.0 ± 0.05	[a]1.7 ± 0.08	[a]1.8 ± 0.08
Saturates	32.3 ± 0.5	31.7 ± 0.3	28.2 ± 0.7
ΣMonounsaturates	43.8 ± 0.7	42.4 ± 0.5	4.0 ± 1.2
ΣPolyunsaturates	23.9 ± 1.2	25.9 ± 0.6	31.8 ± 0.9
Σn-6 PUFAs	21.4 ± 1.1	17.7 ± 0.4	18.2 ± 0.6
Σn-3 PUFAs	2.4 ± 0.2	8.2 ± 0.4	13.5 ± 0.5
Ratio of n-6 to n-3	9.3 ± 0.7	[a]2.2 ± 0.1	[a]1.4 ± 0.05

Source: Modified from Reference 4.

Note. α-LNA = α–linolenic acid, EPA = eicosapentanoic acid, DPA = docosapentanoic acid, DHA = docosahexanoic acid, and PUFA = polyunsaturated fatty acid.

[a]Significantly different from 0% treatment group, $p < 0.05$.

enriched foods. DHA from egg yolk and from mother's milk is very helpful to the infant brain and vascular system development as well as visual acuity.

Although the FA composition of hen eggs can be changed by dietary means, eggs with significant amounts of n-3 PUFAs frequently have an unusual flavor.[18] This can be overcome by using a mixture of commercially available chemical antioxidants and vitamin E.[4] Making the egg flavor as normal as possible is very important if people are going to accept these eggs as food rather than as "medicine."

However, due to the complexity of fatty acids' interactions, sufficient availability of both n-3 and n-6 LCPUFAs, rather than n-3 alone, is required for optimal structural and functional development in infants.[13] Inclusion of 0.2–0.3 percent DHA ensures maximal DHA accretion in the retina of newborn piglets, but cosupplementation with AA is necessary (1) to achieve the same status of blood lipids as that which results from maternal feeding and (2) to prevent any possible imbalance between n-6 and n-3 FAs.[19] One issue that has not been resolved is the origin of DHA and AA for infant neural development.[20] Hence, additional study should be undertaken on whether infants should be dependent on dietary sources before adopting routine use of LCPUFA. Another question concerns the quantity of supplement. In a previous study,[4] we found that eggs are obtained with DHA of 81 and 87 mg/egg by feeding hens diets containing 10 and 20 percent ground flaxseed, which resulted in no significantly different DHA composition between the 10 and 20 percent flax groups (Table 12.2). This result leads to the question of why the concentration change of DHA eggs is not linear to the amount of flax added. It is possible that eggs may have a saturation curve for the maximum absorption of DHA from diet, which might be related to the metabolism of DHA in chickens. Further study needs to be done in order to determine the most efficient quantity of supplementation and to obtain an optimum n-6 to n-3 ratio as well.

References

1. Horrocks, L.A., and Yeo, Y.K. Health benefits of docosahexanoic acid. Pharmacol Res 1999;40:211–25.
2. Van Elswyk, M.E. Comparison of n-3 fatty acid sources in laying hen rations for improvement of whole egg nutritional quality: a review. Br J Nutr 1997;78(suppl. 1):S61–S69.
3. Macrae, R., Robinson, R.K., and Sadler, M.J. Fatty acids. In Encyclopaedia of Food Science, Food Technology, and Nutrition, vol. 3. London; San Diego: Academic Press, 1993, pp. 1741–59.
4. Ferrier, L.K., Caston, L.J., Leeson, S., Squires, J., Weaver, B.J., and Holub, B.J. Alpha-linolenic acid– and docosahexanoic acid–enriched eggs from hens fed flaxseed: influence on blood lipids and platelet phospholipid fatty acids in humans. Am J Clin Nutr 1995;62:81–86.
5. Farrell, D.J. Enrichment of hen eggs with n-3 long-chain fatty acids and evaluation of enriched eggs in humans. Am J Clin Nutr 1996;68:538–44.
6. Horrocks, L.A., and Yeo, Y.K. Docosahexanoic acid-enriched foods: production and effects on blood lipids. Lipids 1999;34(suppl.):S313.
7. Herber, S.M., and Van Elswyk, M.E. Dietary marine algae promote efficient deposition of n-3 fatty acids for the production of enriched shell eggs. Poult Sci 1996;75:1501–7.
8. Barclay, W., Abril, R., Abril, P., Weaver, C., and Ashford, A. Production of docosahexanoic acid from microalgae and its benefits for use in animal feed. World Rev Nutr Diet 1998;83:61–76.
9. William, B. World Rev Nutr Diet 1998;83:61–76.
10. Abril, R., and Barclay, W. Production of docosahexanoic acid-enriched poultry eggs and meat using an algae-based feed ingredient. World Rev Nutr Diet 1998;83:77–88.
11. Crawford, M.A. The role of essential fatty acids in neural development: implications for perinatal nutrition. Am J Clin Nutr 1993;57:703S–709S.
12. Crawford, M.A. Placental delivery of arachidonic and docosahexanoic acids: implications for the lipid nutrition of preterm infants. Am J Clin Nutr 2000;71:275–84.
13. Goustard-Langelier, B., Guesnet, P., Durand, G., Antoine, J.M., and Alessandri, J.M. n-3 and n-6 fatty acid enrichment by dietary fish oil and phospholipid sources in brain cortical areas and nonneural tissues of formula-fed piglets. Lipids 1999;34:5–16.
14. Jensen, C.L., Maude, M., Anderson, R.E., and Heird, W.C. Effect of docosahexanoic acid supplementation of lactating women on the fatty acid composition of breast milk lipids and maternal and infant plasma phospholipids. Am J Clin Nutr 2000;71(suppl.):292S–299S.
15. Simopoulos, A.P., and Salem, N., Jr. Egg yolk as a source of long-chain polyunsaturated fatty acids in infant feeding. Am J Clin Nutr 1992;55:411–14.
16. Nair, S.D., Leitch, J.W., Falconer, J., and Garg, M.L. Prevention of cardiac arrhythmia by

dietary (n-3) polyunsaturated fatty acids and their mechanism of action. J Nutr 1997;127:383–93.

17. McLennana, P., Howea, P., Abeywardenaa, M., Mugglib, R., Raederstorffb, D., Manoa, M., Raynera, T., and Heada, R. The cardiovascular protective role of docosahexanoic acid. Eur J Pharmacol 1996;300:83–89.
18. Jiang, Z., and Sim, J.S. Fatty acid modification of yolk lipids and cholesterol lowering eggs. In Egg Uses and Processing Technologies: New Developments, Sim J.S., and Nakai S., eds. Oxon, UK: CAB International, 1994, pp. 349–61.
19. Alessandri, J.M., Goustard, B., Guesnet, P., and Durand, G. Docosahexanoic acid concentrations in retinal phospholipids of piglets fed an infant formula enriched with long-chain polyunsaturated fatty acids: effects of egg phospholipids and fish oils with different ratios of eicosapentanoic acid to docosahexanoic acid. Am J Clin Nutr 1998;67:377–85.
20. Scott, D.T., Janowsky, J.S., Carroll, R.E., Taylor, J.A., Auestad, N., and Montalto, M.B. Formula supplementation with long-chain polyunsaturated fatty acids: are there developmental benefits? Pediatrics 1998;102:e59.

13

The Correlation between Cholesterol Oxidation Products and Eggs

Jennifer J. Ravia
and Ronald R. Watson

INTRODUCTION

Cholesterol has remained the nemesis of coronary heart disease (CHD) and atheroschlerosis for many years. Research has shown, however, that dietary cholesterol is not as potent to serum cholesterol as once thought. While the debate over dietary cholesterol ebbs and flows, oxysterols have become the center of a new debate. Oxysterols include lipid peroxidation products as well as cholesterol oxidation products. Because the cholesterol content of eggs is higher than the lipid content, the cholesterol oxidation products are of more importance. Cholesterol oxidation products include the following:

7α-hydrocholesterol
7β hydrocholesterol
7-ketocholesterol
cholestanetriol
epoxycholesterol
26-hydroxycholesterol
25-hydroxycholesterol

Cholesterol oxidation products (COPs) result from the auto-oxidation of cholesterol in vitro or the metabolic products of cholesterol in vivo. Although foods that provide abundant amounts of cholesterol usually also contain COPs, there is no direct link between cholesterol disappearance and COP creation.[9] The creation of COPs in high amounts is proportional to determining factors such as light exposure, heat application, and storage time. It is now believed that COPs may elevate the risk of heart disease by contributing to atherogenicity and cytotoxicity (cell death). While it is primarily accepted that dietary cholesterol does not directly influence atherosclerosis, COPs are believed to be involved. However, the exact concentration of ingested COPs that could lead to health complications remains unknown.[4]

Health Risks Associated with COPs

COPs are now being suspected of causing a number of cellular and cardiovascular health problems. Factors that support this claim include the ability of COPs to inhibit sterol biosynthesis, cause membrane dysfunction, and increase cellular calcium leading to cell death.[4] The COP known as 25-hydroxycholesterol has been shown to cause damage to the wall of the aorta, thus beginning the atherosclerotic process.[9] Other COPs have the ability to inhibit the activity of HMG-CoA reductase. A decrease in the activity of this enzyme has the effect of disallowing cholesterol biosynthesis by the body. Cholesterol is needed for the structure and rigidity to be maintained within the plasma membrane. With a decrease in cholesterol, COPs can take the place of the cholesterol in the membrane but cannot provide the membranous support offered by cholesterol. This substitution can lead to cytotoxic problems[9] within the membranes of cells and eventually lead to cell death. Cytosolic and free calcium, although not affected by cholesterol, are influenced by COPs. Both cytosolic and free calcium are increased after COP exposure. Increases in intracellular calcium are known to cause cells to autodestruct. Therefore, by a similar mechanism, high levels of COPs may also lead to autodestruction.[6]

Factors Involved in COP Formation

Powdered eggs have been found to be particularly high in COPs.[1] Egg powder as a food ingredient has become increasingly popular for use in pastas and baked goods. Because of this, eggs (fresh and powdered) and foods that contain powdered eggs have been the focus of much COP research. The parameters of packaging, heating, irradiation, and storage provide a wide range of COP concentrations in egg yolk powder.[2] Spray-dried egg yolk powders were found to contain a significantly higher COP concentration at room temperature than at refrigeration temperature.[2] Pasta made with dried eggs has been shown to have significant levels of COPs. Pasta drying methods include heating at 70–90°C for 10 or more hours. These conditions allow for COP formation, and it has been shown that manufacturing does significantly influence COP formation. COP formation may be controlled by monitoring time and temperature during drying.[1] The actual drying process can also have a substantial effect on the amount of COPs formed. Drying via direct heating with gas produces more COPs than drying via indirect heating with electric heat.[3] This difference was also noted after several months of storage but began to decline after the third month. Free radicals formed during the drying process known as NOx (nitric oxide and nitrite) were present in the air of the gas drying environment but not in that of the electric. When NOx was added to the electric heating environment, COP formation increased.[3] It can be deduced that the higher concentration of COPs in the gas-heated drying method can be attributed to NOx formation during that heating process. While storage has the effect of raising COP concentration within certain foods, irradiation has been shown to have a greater effect of COP formation.[9] This difference may be due to the fact that most storage occurs without light exposure.

Cholesterol Oxidation Products in the Serum

Because of their high cholesterol content, eggs have been avoided in an effort to ward off CHD. Both COPs and lipid peroxidation products are present in eggs and other dehydrated foods, but whether or not these compounds can be absorbed by the body is the focus of some recent research. Foods shown to be high in COP concentration were fed in large amounts to a group of people. The relative amounts of COPs in the blood of these individuals were tested prior to administration and postprandial. A definite rise in blood concentration of COPs was observed, but some discrepancy exists in determining how long serum levels remain elevated.[7] The time interval of serum COP elevation may be important in determining the risk of atherogenecity associated with COPs. The highest COP concentration in the blood occured 24 hours after the meal and remained stable for another 24 hours.[7] Also of some interest is the COP route of travel after being absorbed. When a particular COP was labeled and traced throughout the human body, it was found that COPs can travel in serum bound to albumin or lipoproteins as opposed to cholesterol, which is transferred primarily by lipoproteins.[8] Thus, COP transport was shown to thrive in both regular serum as well as serum that is deficient in lipoproteins. COPs are more polar in nature than cholesterol, which may explain their affinity for albumin when lipoproteins are either unavailable or not present in usable quantities. Moreover, COP concentration was markedly greater in lipoprotein deficient serum with or without albumin present.[8] This leads to the conclusion that COPs are more mobile in the body than is cholesterol and thus have more opportunity to cause damage.

Polyunsaturated Fatty Acids

The intermingling of free oxygen and the double bond in cholesterol leave cholesterol vulnerable to oxidation. It has been suggested that the byproduct of polyunsaturated fatty acid (PUFA) oxidation is needed for the initiation of oxidation of cholesterol.[9] This is supported by the notion that PUFAs are likely to be present in large amounts in foods that contain cholesterol. For example, eggs contain a large amount of oleic and linoleic fatty acids. Furthermore, there is an increased risk of cholesterol oxidation via lipid peroxidation either by natural occurring PUFAs or by eggs coming from hens that ate a PUFA-supplemented diet. PUFA damage appears to worsen as degrees of "unsaturation" and chain length increase.[5] Saturated triglycerides as well as long-chain monounsaturated fatty acid (MUFA) yield little or no cholesterol oxides. The peroxy radicals stemming from these PUFAs may be responsible for the attack on cholesterol that yields the COPs. COP formation is enhanced both by the amount of PUFAs in a food as well as the presence of transition metals, such as iron, that can promote oxysterol formation.[9]

Cholesterol Oxidation Products and Food

Because COP concentration in the blood can be influenced by dietary factors, it is important to analyze the COP concentration within the diet. Dehydrated foods such as heat-dried egg yolk powder contain more COPs than fresh foods in general, and fresh eggs do not contain COPs in any more than a trace amount. Zunin et al. reported that when fresh eggs were frozen and stored, no COPs were formed. Baked biscuits and snacks made with egg powder yielded more COP formation than the same foods made with fresh eggs.[4] Water as an ingredient or byproduct of heating in foods seems to inhibit cholesterol oxidation. Foods that exhibit the most surface area tend to have higher levels of COPs. This partially explains the large concentrations of COPs found in powdered eggs.[4] COPs do not usually all show up in one product. Most likely different foods contain different COPs.

The Effects of Antioxidant Administration

Zunin et al. proposed that naturally occurring caretenoids in eggs inhibit COP formation by competing for free radicals.[1] When antioxidants were added to the eggs being dried in a gas-heated environment, there was no significant effect on COP formation. Egg powders from α-tocopherol–supplemented hens had a lower concentration of COPs after heating and during storage. As storage time increased, available α-tocopherol decreased. Though vitamin E appears to be able to decrease the formation of COPs, it has not been shown to prevent cytotoxicity in cells from existing COPs.[6] Studies have shown that vitamin E failed to protect cells from the induced cytotoxic effects of some of the more potent COPs. Vitamin E has been shown to protect against atherosclerotic damage by acting as a preventative antioxidant. However, in the event that COPs have already initiated damage, such as taking over a cell membrane, the time period for preventative maintenance may have expired, leaving vitamin E without the ability to decrease COP concentrations.

Conclusion

Although cholesterol oxidation products have been shown to be absorbed and cause damage within the body, the COP concentration necessary to initiate the damage remains unknown. While fresh foods containing cholesterol have only trace amounts of COPs, foods that have been dehydrated, exposed to light, or stored contain a much higher percentage of COPs. Eggs have been the focus of many studies due to their extensive use in the food industry and high initial amounts of intact cholesterol. Though eggs have numerous health benefits, the presence of COPs could be a disadvantage. This cannot be determined until further research has demonstrated exactly what range of COPs causes harmful effects within the body. Further research is also needed to illustrate the COP concentration differences among foods. Results of research in this nature could provide evidence of the degree of potential damage by eggs as compared with other cholesterol-rich foods. Research has shown no significant evidence of any substances having the ability to halt or hinder COP formation. If COPs are actually found to cause illness, more studies will be needed to search for a substance, antioxidant or otherwise, that has the ability to decrease COP formation. Cholesterol oxidation products have the potential to perform harm within the body, and although it has been shown that COP concentrations are higher in eggs than in most foods, the concentration necessary to threaten health remains unknown.

References

1. Zunin, P., Evangelisti, C., Calcagno, C., and Tiscornia, E. Cholesterol oxidation in dried egg pasta: detecting 7-ketocholesterol content. Cereal Chem 1996;73:691–94.
2. Ahn, D.U., Lee, J.I., Jo, C., and Sell, J.L. Analysis of cholesterol oxides in egg yolk and turkey meat. Poult Sci 1999;78:1060–64.
3. Lai, S., Gray, I., Buckley, D.J., and Kelly, P.M. Influence of free radicals and other factors on formation of cholesterol oxidation products in spray-dried whole egg. J Agric Food Chem 1995;43:1127–31.
4. Zunin, P., Evangelisti, F., Caboni, M.F., Penazzi, G., Lercker, G., and Tiscornia, E. Cholesterol oxidation in baked foods containing fresh and powdered eggs. J Food Sci 1995;60:913–17.
5. Li, S.X., Cherian, G., and Sim, J.S. Cholesterol oxidation in egg yolk powder during storage and heating as affected by dietary oils and tocopherol. J Food Sci 1996;61:721–25.
6. Zhou, Q., Wasowicz, E., and Kummerow, F. Failure of vitamin E to protect cultured human arterial smooth muscle cells against oxysterol induced cytotoxicity. J Am Coll Nutr 1995;14:169–75.
7. Emanuel, H.A., Hassel, C.A., Addis, P.B., Bergman, S.D., and Zavoral, J.H. Plasma cholesterol oxidation products (oxysterols) in human subjects fed a meal rich in oxysterols. J Food Sci 1991;56:843–47.
8. Lin, C.Y., and Morel, D.W. Distribution of oxysterols in human serum: characterization of 25-hydroxycholesterol association with serum albumin. Nutr Biochem 1995;6:618–25.
9. Paniangvait, P., King, A.J., Jones, A.D., and German, B.G. Cholesterol oxides in foods of animal origin. J Food Sci 1995;60:1159–73.

Section 3

Eggs and Disease: Health Promotion

14

Whole Eggs: The Magic Bullet?

H.L. "Sam" Queen

mág•ic búl•let, "something that cures or remedies without causing harmful side effects."

WHOLE EGGS: THE MAGIC BULLET?

Consider for a moment the following hypothetical event. Someone hands you the magic bullet for heart disease, which is then injected into a dear family member who has high cholesterol and grossly narrowed arteries. This magic bullet would enable your loved one to overcome the heart- and life-threatening consequences of such a scenario, with relatively little effort, low cost, and no unpleasant side effects. What if that magic bullet was actually (gasp!) an egg?

Whole eggs have long been maligned as a cause of high serum cholesterol and heart disease, mostly because they contain substantial amounts of fat and cholesterol. Strangely, this attitude has been taken by health authorities without ever studying whole eggs directly. Recommendations to limit daily consumption were initially based on cholesterol content and epidemiological evidence, such as Ancel Keys' Seven Country Study.[1] Over the next 30 or so years this impression was supported by a continuous deluge of animal and human studies, which heart authorities contended was indisputable evidence of cause and effect.[2] So certain were authorities that the cause of heart disease had been found that they formed the National Cholesterol Education Program (NCEP), fully expecting (through education) to eradicate heart disease by the year 2000. Well, 2000 has come and gone, fewer eggs are being consumed as planned, but the problem remains just about as it was.

Looking back, nearly all of the early egg studies had serious flaws. They were primarily performed in metabolic wards and cages—settings that were far removed from the free living conditions experienced by most people and animals. Adding to the unnatural design, the test diets generally consisted of dried egg products rich in oxidized cholesterol rather than whole eggs that were free of oxidized products. So the outcome, while convincing to many scientists, fell far short of typifying the conditions under which eggs are normally consumed by people.

Recent studies that you'll read about throughout this book have lightened the charge against eggs. Nevertheless, the strength and weight of past evidence continues to discourage researchers from proposing a direct clinical trial of whole eggs. Adding to the resistance, institutional review boards generally take the attitude that feeding whole eggs to people would be cruel and inhumane, given the "facts." So scientists who wish to examine the relationship of eggs and heart disease have taken to evaluating long-term heart and diet patterns of free-living individuals. They compare the cardiovascular endpoints of people who eat eggs against endpoints of those who eat few to no eggs per day.

Two such examinations in which this has been done are the Nurses Health Study[3] (involving more than 80,000 female subjects) and the Health Professionals Study[4] (involving more than 40,000 male subjects). To the general dismay of those who have advocated fewer eggs per day, no definitive link could be made between whole egg consumption patterns, higher serum cholesterol, and heart attack risk. Other major studies have resulted in similar conclusions (see chap. 8). This lack of support for past recommendations has prompted the new conclusion that eggs are neither a risk factor nor a cause of heart attack.

With the recent overturning of the past indictment of whole eggs, the lever needed to lobby for a direct, clinical trial is now in place, just waiting for someone to apply the pressure. For those who are still concerned about safety, it is suggested they review the data of cohorts within the previously mentioned studies and compare the people who ate the most eggs with those who ate the least. Since the bottom line shows no difference in heart disease risk among egg eaters and non–egg eaters, it is logical that cohorts will be found within each group that fared far better and far worse. The differences are likely to be accounted for not just by the number or frequency of eggs eaten but by the differences in genetics and the accompanying diet and lifestyle choices. Understanding the differences may make all the difference in determining whether you think of eggs as the problem or the magic bullet.

Searching for That Magic Bullet: Would We Recognize It If We Saw It?

Let's consider our hypothetical event in which you've received a magic bullet for your loved one. If the potion lived up to its claim, what immediate change would you expect in serum cholesterol level and appearance and makeup of arterial lesions? Indeed, an immediate physical change would be seen in the lesions. Whether the change was immediately for the better would be debatable.

The change seen in serum cholesterol would be less debatable. You would, of course, see a rise in serum cholesterol, since it would be exiting the lesion and entering the bloodstream. Although this initial rise would logically be a sign of success, researchers and clinicians have never regarded any rise in cholesterol as a good thing. A rise in cholesterol from any challenge—even the magic bullet—would be regarded by them as a bad thing. Given this flawed perception, it is possible (and likely) that science has stumbled onto the magic bullet many times without realizing it.

Supposing again that eggs were the magic bullet, what changes in serum cholesterol would you expect over an extended period when eggs were consumed by free-living people who began with a slight baseline elevation? Logic tells us that serum cholesterol would rise even more, especially at first, as the bloodstream is at the confluence of cholesterol entering via the diet and cholesterol that's being released from the material that makes up arterial lesions. However, as the lesions regressed in size and severity due to this magic bullet, and as the excess cholesterol got redistributed, the serum level would later return to baseline or below.

To evaluate the possibility that eggs may bring about a cholesterol curve that mimics the magic bullet effect, a stair-step study of free-living people was carried out in the late 1970s by Elliott,[5] who looked first at the combined effect of egg feeding on serum cholesterol and LCAT (the enzyme responsible for esterification, which packs more cholesterol into high-density lipoprotein [HDL] than might otherwise occur). The study, involving an isocaloric substitution of four eggs per day, was carried out for 12 weeks in 15 test subjects who served as their own controls, 12 of whom completed the study. Beginning with the 5th week, the test subjects added a daily supplement of 2 g of vitamin C to the egg regimen. On the 9th week the test subjects added regular exercise to the vitamin C and egg regimen. Too, since cholesterol can only exit the body through the intestinal tract, only those people who reported having two or more bowel movements per day were chosen for the study. To assist in keeping cholesterol and bile from being reabsorbed, a high-fiber diet was also required, and all participants agreed to adjust calories and exercise so as to maintain a constant body weight throughout the study period.

Total serum cholesterol rose at first in all participants, as anticipated, in response to the increase in egg consumption. By week 12 the cholesterol level had subsided in all but one person to a level that was either equal to or less than the baseline reading. In the lone exception, serum cholesterol went up and stayed up and was accompanied by failure of the LCAT enzyme to respond (rise). This scenario was indeed consistent with what you might expect from administering any hypothetical magic bullet under similar diet and lifestyle circumstances. Yet, because the study involved whole eggs, because it produced a rise in serum cholesterol early in the study as experts anticipated, because it involved so few people, and perhaps because it failed to get reported in a key heart journal, the findings were not considered remarkable. Nevertheless, the study offers a model of the changes you might expect in serum cholesterol in response to any magic bullet that uses cholesterol to fight cholesterol.

A second common flaw in searching for the magic bullet comes from the fact that science tends to look at data from the disease perspective while ignoring the health perspective. An example is the discovery of a specialized protein that brought about the need for this discussion and that is largely responsible for the magic bullet effect of eggs, *apoprotein E* (apo E).

Apoprotein E

Let's begin with a little background. Apoproteins comprise the major protein components of all lipoproteins. A search in 1963 for the cause of abetalipoproteinemia (an unusual condition characterized by a very low total serum cholesterol and neurological symptoms) revealed that there are five major apoproteins, known today as apo A, B, C, D, and E.[6] All five are in short supply in that condition, which suggested that a deficiency of these proteins is not a good thing. Further work soon revealed that apoproteins perform the following basic functions:

1. They assist in the maturation process of lipoproteins.
2. They serve as cofactors for the enzymes that promote lipid metabolism (i.e., lipoprotein lipase and LCAT) by providing a suitable lipid interface upon which the enzymes can work.
3. They participate in the cell-to-cell distribution and redistribution of cholesterol, thereby serving as precursors for steroid production.
4. They play a significant role in escorting cholesterol not just through, but out of, the body.

Apo E is fundamental to the mechanism by which eggs, given the right circumstances, may impart a magic bullet effect. Apo E is associated with very low-density lipoprotein (VLDL) and two unique HDL particles (HDL1 and HDLc), which are not normally included in routine HDL testing. The two particles contain far more cholesterol than is contained in the HDL that's normally measured. The usual testing procedure, performed by the heparin/manganese precipitin method, measures only the cholesterol attributed to HDL2 + HDL3. The cholesterol measured in HDL1 and HDLc (derived mostly from eating eggs and butter) shows up in the total cholesterol reading.

This difference is *quite* significant, as HDL1 and HDLc are perhaps the most important particles for redistributing cholesterol collected from areas of high concentration for delivery to where it is either needed or excreted. This *reverse cholesterol transport* system begins with apo A, which is responsible for picking up cholesterol from areas of high concentration and loading it aboard HDL3 and HDL2. Once aboard, the LCAT enzyme esterifies the cholesterol so that it can be tightly packed and stored in the triglyceride-rich core. HDL's tightly packed cholesterol load can then be delivered either to the liver for excretion or redistributed to areas where cholesterol is needed. This latter benefit, which is sometimes seen as a means by which the arterial intima accumulates too much cholesterol, can largely be attributed to apo E, the key apoprotein of egg-induced HDL.

Early studies of apo E by the research team of Dr. Robert Mahley at the Gladstone Foundation in San Francisco revealed that diets high in eggs and other cholesterol sources brought about a rise in serum cholesterol in the majority of his subjects.[7] While the cholesterol response was initially looked upon with suspicion, it was nevertheless found to be due to a rise in a cholesterol-rich HDL particle that differed from the usual HDL. Apo E accounted for the altered HDL particle and served a potentially helpful role in disposing of the additional cholesterol load.[8] As a ligand, or binding agent, it tended to target receptors prevalent in the brain, the nervous system, steroid-producing glands, and the liver's catabolic pool.[9]

Upon seeing this reality, it became clear how apo E was designed to work together with apo A to our benefit. The process has been extensively explained,[10] but it largely occurs in this way: Apo A picks up cholesterol from areas of high cholesterol concentration, after which apo E docks with certain tissues so that the cholesterol load can be delivered to where it is needed or to where the excess can be excreted (where cholesterol is delivered to the liver's catabolic pool).[11]

When apo E was first discovered and understood, the health benefit credited to it seemed sufficiently clear, enough that by the mid-1980s many credible scientists saw it as playing a positive role in the reversal of atherosclerosis.[12] It was at this point that the health perspective got replaced by a disease perspective, due mostly to the fact that the receptors for the so-called bad cholesterol of low-density lipoprotein (LDL) tended to also show affinity for cholesterol delivered by apo E. Since arterial disease was being associated with oxidized LDL, then apo E was lumped under the same "bad" label. Being disease oriented, authorities then turned their focus totally away from the health-promoting function of apo E and toward the bad. Rather than acknowledging that 80 percent of people benefited from apo E, doctors warned that it raised the risk for developing type III hyperlipoproteinemia (a rare condition) and risked making type II and type IV hyperlipoproteinemia worse (even more rare). From that point forward, without being shown due respect for their benefits, eggs and apo E were considered either bad or suspect.

While Mahley's research team could not control how authorities used its findings, it nevertheless continued to look at the potential benefit from apo E in areas other than heart health. For starters, the researchers were impressed with the fact that the sciatic nerve of a rat had the propensity to mend itself when severed and that the mending process was accompanied by a massive accumulation of cholesterol at the site of injury. Quite naturally, they and other apo E enthusiasts began wondering what role cholesterol played in the mending process of nerves and if apo E might be responsible for directing cholesterol to the injured site. Mahley's team had, after all, just revealed that the macrophages that emerged following injury were a primary endogenous source of apo E.

Research into the process of nerve repair and remyelination revealed that apo E from macrophages that arises following injury serves to sequester the axon debris along with membrane cholesterol, fatty acids, and other lipids.[13] The sequestered cholesterol is then metabolized to pregnenolone and progesterone, just as it is in the gonads and the adrenal glands, which provide the steroidal effect needed to regenerate and remyelinate the nerve. Among neurologists, this finding was big stuff, as it suggested that remyelination and repair of human nerves might be possible by learning how to express apo E to its maximum. To answer this question, Mahley's research team pointed to earlier work where the team had shown that the addition of four to six eggs per day to the diet of six healthy men and women volunteers had brought about a six-fold increase in the expression of apo E. This finding caused apo E researchers to conclude two important points:

1. Apo E is highly active in the redistribution of cholesterol.
2. Adding four to six eggs per day to the diet increases the activity of apo E up to six-fold and thereby improves the mechanism by which nerves are repaired and myelin is regenerated. (Fig. 14.1 lists some factors other than eggs involved in apo E biosynthesis.)

The health benefits that can be credited to the redistribution process extend far beyond rebuilding and remyelinating nerves. Here is one example of which I have intimate knowledge.

In the early 1970s, I worked in a large clinical laboratory, performing bicarbonate determinations with the historically important Van Slyke Apparatus. The Van Slyke Apparatus

Apo E Biosynthesis

Apo E biosynthesis is stimulated by thyroid hormone.[1] By the same token, receptors for apo E serve to facilitate thyroid hormone uptake into a variety of tissues.[2] Thus, thyroid activity may serve as a marker of apo E activity. A low level may negatively influence the production of apo E. Based on this observation, researchers confirmed that the level of insulin is not only related inversely to thyroid function but also to apo E biosynthesis.[3] Not surprising, then, a diet based on sugar and white flour will stunt apo E output, while (as Mahley's group had demonstrated) a diet based on eggs and butter tends to stimulate production of apo E the most.

Apo E is also synthesized by the liver and macrophages following ingestion of a fatty, sterol-rich meal and during the healthy acute inflammatory response. Conversely, either a fat-free diet or chronic inflammation (or both) tends to depress the total output of apo E.[4]

1. Vandanbrouck, Y., et al., The modulation of apolipoprotein E gene expression by 3, 3'-5-triiodothyronine in HepG2 cells occurs at transcriptional and post-transcriptional levels, Eur J Biochem, September 1, 1994;224(2):463–71.
2. Benvenga, S., Cahnmann, H.J., and Robbins, J., Characterization of thyroid hormone binding to apolipoprotein-E: localization of the binding site in the exon 3-coded domain, Endocrinol, September 1993;133(3):1300–5.
3. Ogbonna, G., Theriault, A., and Adeli, K., Hormonal regulation of human apolipoprotein E gene expression in HepG2 cells, Int J Biochem, May 1993;25(5):635–40.
4. Werb, Z., et al., The cell and molecular biology of apolipoprotein E synthesis by microphages, Ciba Found Symp 1986;118:155–71.

Figure 14.1. Biosynthesis.

held about 600 ml liquid mercury in a "closed" system. In the normal process of using the apparatus, laboratory workers were exposed to mercury vapors and liquid mercury that spilled from leaky stopcocks. After far too many technologists had either died or become seriously ill, OSHA came to the aid of the laboratory staff by requiring that the Van Slyke be used thereafter only under a vented hood. Today, it is seldom used at all.

As for me, I suffered from brain stem deterioration due to significant chronic exposure to mercury and was not expected to live. My recovery was credited largely to the practice of eating six eggs per day, also including a regimen of daily aerobic exercise, good bowel function, a high fiber diet, and supplementation with an ultramegadose vitamin C, based on the knowledge I'd gained from what others have researched. In retrospect, I believe my recovery can most accurately be credited to apo E stimulated by the regular consumption of eggs. In contrast, people with this condition who do not eat eggs generally fail to survive.

Some other established health benefits are the building of steroid hormones and the making of bile. In the process, the shuttlelike mechanism credited to apoproteins allows heavy metals to be picked up and removed from metal-sensitive brain and nerve cells. For those brave souls who can bring themselves to accept the reality that a rise in cholesterol can be useful, the benefit comes from the redistribution of cholesterol from areas of excess to areas of need. Just such a scenario is what you would expect in anyone who had been given a magic bullet not only for cholesterol-laden arteries but also for nerves affected by toxic pesticides and metals.

The desired outcome, however, would not likely be seen in someone who failed to follow the rules for good cholesterol turnover:

1. Consume sufficient vitamin C each day to complete the synthesis of bile.
2. Engage in regular exercise.
3. Eat a high-fiber diet.
4. Have 2 or more formed bowel movements per day.

We consider this "earning the right to eat eggs."

All People Do Not Receive Equal Benefit from Apo E or Eggs

Although we come from the same conceptual design, we are all different. This difference, which is clearly reflected in genetics, also results from factors that are mostly under our control, such as diet, lifestyle, stress response, choice of profession, and environmental exposures. Collectively, these and differences that may not be so obvious help explain the mechanism by which eggs can be beneficial to some people but not to others. Of greatest consideration, however, especially where apo E is involved, is genetics.

Genetics plays a major role as to whether you can expect to receive the magic bullet effect from eating eggs without additional special effort. It also goes a long way toward determining if you will be more or less susceptible to coronary artery disease (CAD) or Alzheimer's disease, which tend to occur together (although arterial disease often kills a person before the Alzheimer aspect can manifest).[14] Apo E can play a protective role, and a deficiency leads to the most severe cases of arterial disease. Yet, as others have pointed out, an increase may lead to both arterial disease and Alzheimer's disease.[15] To help unravel the mystery for how the latter might happen, and how you might respond in a positive way to offset unfavorable genetics and outcomes, the following discussion is offered.

Understanding the Apo E/Egg Connection

Eggs stimulate apo E activity in accordance with your inherited phenotype, and it is the genes that make up the phenotype that determine the good or bad outcome from eating eggs. Genetically, the genes for apo E appear as either apo E-2, E-3, or E-4. Each person inherits two copies of the gene, one from each parent, resulting in six possible phenotypes:

- apo E-2/2
  apo E-2/3
  apo E-2/4
- apo E-3/3
  apo E-3/4
- apo E-4/4

People who are most likely to derive the magic bullet effect are those with either the apo E-2/3 or 3/3 phenotypes. The following discussion provides background information needed to develop a plan so that every person can experience the magic bullet effect if he or she is willing to work at it.

Apo E-2

Some combination of genes involving apo E-2 is found in about 10–13 percent of the population and tends to offer the most protection against Alzheimer's but less protection against arterial disease. Yet even that risk is small. About 1 in 1,000 people who carry the E-2/2 phenotype develops a risk to arterial disease from type III hyperlipoproteinemia (due to reduced affinity for binding to receptors in the liver). A second cohort of people with apo E-2/2 tends to have a great risk for infection, angina, and high blood pressure and thus may have a higher risk for arterial disease.

Apo E-3

The apo E-3 gene, positioned in three of the six phenotypes, apo E-3/2, E-3/3, and E-3/4, is the ancestral allele isoform that most people have, which helps protect against arterial disease as well as Alzheimer's disease. Nearly 80 percent of people have inherited at least one gene of apo E-3 from their two parents, and it is this 80 percent of the population that can benefit most from eating eggs. Again, however, the tendency by authorities has been to impose restrictions on all egg eaters rather than to look at how to improve the health of that 20 percent of the population who carry the health-sensitive apo E-2 and E-4 isoforms.

Apo E-4

The apo E-4 gene, existing in one of three combinations (either E-4/4, E-2/4, or E-3/4), predisposes people to Alzheimer's disease and CAD. Although not everyone who has these phenotypes gets Alzheimer's or CAD, 95 percent of Alzheimer's people carry at least 1 allele for E-4.[16] With regard to treatment, the standard drug used to treat Alzheimer's disease works best on people who are free of the apo E-4 allele.

Apo E-4 also predisposes people to atherosclerosis and to a variety of hyperlipidemias, including the potentially fatal type II hyperlipoproteinemia, which is generally a more serious condition in those people who carry an apo E-4 gene from each parent and who express the apo E-4/4 phenotype. To assess the total heart disease contribution of apo E-4, regardless of the lipid phenotype, a group of Italian researchers looked at 106 young European adults who had a history of myocardial infarction.[17] True to form, the presence of one or more apo E-4 alleles demonstrated (with a 95 percent confidence interval) a strong independent predictor of adverse events, with each allele raising the risk for heart attack (in people over age 65) by a factor of 2.84. A similar relationship could be found in a study of the people of Saudi Arabia.[18]

Looking further at the general contribution of apo E isoforms to arterial disease, researchers have recently demonstrated—using CT scans—that in people bearing apo E-4 there is a far greater extent of coronary artery calcification than in people who carry other apo E alleles.[19]

Apo E-4 may further contribute to a rise in coronary events and CAD severity through producing more free radicals than its apo E counterparts.[20] Oxidized LDL, for instance, is more prevalent in people who carry one or more apo E-4 alleles than in other people. The excess free radicals generated by apo E-4 can be accounted for by the excesses of nitric oxide produced by the arginine substrate and from failure to bind with and extract heavy metals due to lack of cysteine. (See Table 14.1 for a description of the amino acid differences in apo E.)

The amino acid differences in the various apo E isoforms give some hints as to why some phenotypes are more and less protective than others. Knowing these differences may also help in developing a strategy for improving the outcome of eating eggs no matter what the person's apo E phenotype.

Table 14.1. Amino acid differences among the three Apo E isoforms and their relationship to Alzheimer's disease and coronary artery disease (CAD) risk

Apoprotein	Cysteine	Arginine	Alzheimer's risk	CAD risk
apo E-2	2	0	Lowest Risk	Average Risk
apo E-3	1	1	Average Risk	Lowest Risk
apo E-4	0	2	Highest Risk	Highest Risk

Problems with E-4

Degeneration of cells of the nerves, brain, and arteries tend to occur most readily with an apo E-4/4 phenotype. This can largely be explained by the substitution of arginine for cysteine on codon 112 and 158 that characterize the various apo E phenotypes.[21] (Codons are bases located on a strand of DNA that direct the incorporation of a specific amino acid into a polypeptide chain.) Cysteine, directed by codon 112 in the apo E-2 and apo E-3 alleles, is characterized by the conspicuous presence of a terminal $^{-}$SH group that allows it to latch onto a heavy metal or pesticide during its interchange with the target tissue.[23] (Thiols bearing the $^{-}$SH group bind to portions of any compound that is deficient in electrons—making them good conjugates of heavy metals and pesticides.) In contrast, apo E-4 is absent of cysteine and thereby lacks the necessary $^{-}$SH group to latch onto heavy metals and select pesticides. So wherever heavy metals or pesticides are causing damage—such as in the brain, the nerves, the adrenal glands, or the arteries—the cysteine portion of apo E present in egg-induced HDL serves to remove the metal and protect the tissue site. The substitution of arginine for cysteine in apo E-4 allows heavy metals to do damage where they might otherwise be neutralized and extracted from affected tissues.

Arginine, directed by codon 158 on apo E-4 and E-3, provides its own beneficial role by serving as substrate for nitric oxide (NO), an acidic free radical that serves both as an antibacterial and as a smooth muscle relaxant needed to control blood pressure and prevent spasms of the arteries and other NO-sensitive tissues. However, when arginine is present in excess, such as would most likely occur in someone who was homozygous for apo E-4, and accompanied by an excess of the enzyme that induces its synthesis (iNOS), NO becomes a liability rather than a benefit due to excessive acidity and free radical output. So the differences in amino acid content of the various apo E isoforms help to account for why the cysteine-rich apo E-2 and E-3 isoforms are more protective against brain metals and why arginine-rich apo E-4 might raise the risk for Alzheimer's, lower the risk for metal toxicity, cause early-onset arterial disease, and result in a higher risk for brain damage following a stroke (where acidity becomes the determinant of damage). Reactive oxygen species (ROS), for instance, are known to be produced in greater quantity in an acidic environment than in a more alkaline environment.[24]

From this relationship it is reasonable that people with E-4, lacking the metal-binding cysteine, are the people who may want to limit egg consumption until a health program can be tailored to fit their needs. Otherwise, these are the people who react first to low-level exposure to toxic metals and who tend to develop Alzheimer's disease where heavy metals become a precipitating factor. In this scenario there is no cysteine to bind with mercury and other heavy metals. The buildup of brain acidity from the NO intensifies both the metal's reactivity and the brain's susceptibility to damage. In addition, because of the weakened interactions of apo E-4 for tau-protein (which helps prevent Alzheimer's disease by regulating the stability of microtubulin), apo E-4 further promotes Alzheimer's disease by destabilizing the microtubulin.

Apo E-2, being heavily endowed with the sulfhydryl-rich cysteine, binds readily with heavy metals but (lacking the arginine substrate) fails to produce sufficient NO production to help fight infection and to allow for proper smooth muscle relaxation. The lack of NO may also fail to stimulate sufficient lipase needed to metabolize triglyceride fats, which may largely account for the heightened risk for glucose intolerance seen in people who express the apo E-2/2 phenotype and who consume eggs in quantity. For these people to receive the magic bullet effect, they need to have a program tailored for them.

Apo E-3, carrying one molecule each of both cysteine and arginine, tends to produce the best overall protection against a variety of health conditions where cysteine and arginine may play a role.

Apo E-4, as stated earlier, offers no protection against heavy metals, which have been implicated as an initiating factor not only in Alzheimer's and CAD but also in many toxicities and other diseases as well. Fortunately, it occurs in only 3–10 percent of the population. Yet people who carry one or more apo E-4 alleles account for more than 70 percent of the people with Alzheimer's, making it a very high risk factor.[25,26,27] While apo E-2/4 and apo E-3/4 slightly raise the risk of Alzheimer's, people with E-4/4 are at the highest risk, especially after experiencing a head injury. This makes sense since apo E activity is known to rise in response to macrophages that naturally accompany nerve and brain injuries. While the purpose is to restore health to the injured site, the increase in apo E activity in people who express arginine-rich apo E-4 results in an excess of NO. The acidic nature of NO causes a serious drop in the threshold for when the "tangles" of microtubulin familiar to Alzheimer's patients become evident.

For People Who Express the Apo E-2/2, E-2/4, E-3/4, or E-4/4 Phenotype, What Chance Do They Have of Experiencing the Magic Bullet Effect?

For those lucky ones who've inherited E-2/3 or E-3/3, they have the best chance to experience the magic bullet effect. People in the other groups will have more difficulty. Supplementation will improve their odds.

While this question begs for a quick and easy answer, the research in this area is lacking. Yet the facts suggest that a strategy can be implemented with some anticipated success. If you have inherited E-2/2, E-2/4, E-3/4, or E-4/4, the following steps might be considered to improve outcome.

Apo E-2/2

Focus on foods that are rich in arginine, which is lacking with this phenotype and is necessary to provide NO. You might also consider supplementing with arginine in accordance with the following conservative dosage schedule of 500 mg at bedtime for a 150-pound person.

Apo E-2/4, E-3/4, and E-4/4

Focus on foods that are rich in glutathione, such as asparagus, lamb, veal, parsley, and avocado.[29] Otherwise, you might consider supplementing L-glutathione in accordance with the dosage schedule of 300 mg per day for a 150-pound person, per egg per day. (Glutathione is safer than supplementing with cysteine because cysteine given as an amino acid may be neurotoxic.) Some intestinal absorption occurs, but maximum absorption occurs in the oral cavity across oral mucosa.[28] Thus, you might mix glutathione powder in water and drink it slowly.

Conclusion

While the average person may have difficulty altering their long-held perceptions, whole eggs, by stimulating a rise in apo E activity, possess the potential for serving as the magic bullet for not only preventing heart disease but also reversing it. The outcome, however, whether good or bad, depends first and foremost on whether the person has earned the right to eat eggs. If this person is not following the basic steps required for good cholesterol turnover, then he or she certainly hasn't earned the right and is not likely to get the magic bullet effect no matter his or her apo E phenotype. This person should probably limit egg intake to no more than one per day.

For those who comply with the rules for good cholesterol turnover as outlined in the Elliott study, the clinician might then award them with a prescription to test for both an apo E phenotype and an apo E activity level. With this data in hand and a cohort of highly cooperative test subjects, a pilot study could then be conducted with relative safety regarding the effects on the arteries of a free-living group of men and women expressing either the apo E-2/3 or E-3/3 phenotype who volunteer to eat whole eggs daily and in quantity. They would predictably experience the magic bullet effect.

There are other caveats that might be considered before doing any study that could skew results. At the Institute for Health Realities, for instance, we do a very extensive blood analysis before our health coach team offers any advice because there are so many other factors that need to be addressed if health is the ultimate goal. If this is done, the information provided in this chapter begs for a second study of people who bear either the apo E-2/2, E-2/4, E-3/4, or E-4/4 phenotype, who would predictably have difficulty in experiencing the magic bullet effect. The findings would help determine just how many eggs they can eat safely and to what extent that they too can participate in gaining the benefits.

For the person with the apo E-2/2 phenotype, who has difficulty metabolizing fatty acids due to reduced lipase activity, the research team might make certain beforehand that he or she qualifies as per the requirements for apo E biosynthesis (see Figure 14.1) and perhaps even supplement with the lipase enzyme. Having screened the subjects adequately, researchers might further supplement their program with a nominal daily dosage of arginine for the purpose of supplying the missing nitric oxide.

For the person bearing an apo E-4 phenotype the project could be expanded to include supplementation with reduced L-glutathione to provide a readily functional source of intracellular, sulfhydryl binding.

It seems logical, given the evidence, that whole eggs offer the perfect magic bullet not only for unclogging arteries and handling the infections that often associate with arterial lesions but also for removing heavy metals from the brain and nervous system, for reducing the risk for Alzheimer's disease, and for reducing smooth muscle spasms in people with angina and high blood pressure. Even people with the most troublesome apo E phenotypes can benefit. The key to this level of success from eating whole eggs, however, would largely rest on the relationship between the health care provider, whose role it is to test and advise, and the person who seeks the magic bullet, whose role it is to work diligently toward earning the right to eat them.

Dedication

This chapter is dedicated to three people who have played an important role in our understanding of egg nutrition.

- H.B. Wallace, my mentor and close friend who pioneered the egg industry and who now administers the Wallace Research Foundation.
- The late Blanton Smith of Nashville, Tennessee, who bravely and openly placed a full page ad in the Wall Street Journal stating, "There is no scientific evidence, whatsoever, that eating eggs increases your risk to heart disease." While a retraction to the statement was forced in a U.S. district court, I was impressed that those who testified to the contrary could never prove that the statement was wrong.
- Fred Kummerow, Ph.D., of the Burnside Research Laboratory, University of Illinois, Urbana/Champaign, who provided the initial key testimony on behalf of eggs in the now famous Egg Trial and who continues to look at the many causal factors in heart disease.

References

1. Keys, A., ed. Coronary heart disease in seven countries. Circulation 1970;4(Suppl. I): I–211.
2. Lipid Research Clinics (LRC) Program. The LRC Coronary Primary Prevention Trial Results: II. The relationship of reduction in incidence of coronary heart disease to cholesterol lowering. JAMA 1984;251:365–74.
3. Hu, F.B., Stampfer, M.J., Manson, J.E., Rimm, E., Colditz, G.A., Rosner, B.A., Hennekens, C.H. and Willett, W.C. Dietary fat intake and the risk of coronary heart disease in women. NEJM 1997;337:1491–99.
4. Ascherio, A., Rimm, E.B., Giovanucci, E.L., Spiegelman, D., Stampfer, M.J., and Willett, W.C.. Dietary fat and risk of coronary heart disease in men: cohort follow up study in the United States. BMJ 1996;313:84–90.
5. Elliott, H.C. Lecithin-cholesterol acyltransferase (LCAT) response to dietary cholesterol loading. Clin Chem 1978;24: 2068.
6. Levy, R.I. Cholesterol, lipoproteins, apoproteins, and heart disease: Present status and future prospects. Clin Chem 1981;27(5):653–62.
7. Mahley, R.W., et al. Alterations in human high density lipoproteins, with or without increased plasma-cholesterol, induced by diets high in cholesterol. Lancet, Oct. 14, 1978;2:807–9.
8. Mahley, R.W. Atherogenic hyperlipoproteinemia. The cellular and molecular biology of plasma lipoproteins altered by dietary fat and cholesterol. Med Clin N Am 1982;66(2):375–402.
9. Elshourbagy, N.A., Liao, W.S., Mahley, R.W., and Taylor, J.M. Apo-E mRNA is abundant in the brain and adrenals as well as in the liver, and is present in other peripheral tissues of rats and marmosets. Proc Natl Acad Sci, Jan. 1985;82:203–7.

10. Queen, H.L. Reversing chemical- or neurotoxin-induced damage to the brain and nervous system. Health Talk, Sept. 1990;9(2):9–16.
11. Koo, C., Innerarity, T.L., and Mahley, R.W. Obligatory role of cholesterol and apoprotein E in the formation of large cholesterol-enriched and receptor-active HDL. J Bio Chem, 1985;260(22):11934–43.
12. Getz, G.S., Mazzone, T., Soltys, P., and Bates, S.R. Atherosclerosis and apoprotein E. An enigmatic relationship, Arch Pathol Lab Med, 1988;112(10):1048–55.
13. Boyles, J.K., Zoellner, C.D., Anderson, L.J., Kosik, L.M., Pitas, R.E., Weisgraber, K.H., Hui, D.Y., Mahley, R.W., Gebicke-Haerter, P.J. Ignatius, M.J., and Shooter, E.M. A role for apo E, apo-A-1, and LDL receptors in cholesterol transport during regeneration and remyelination of the rat sciatic nerve, J Clin Invest, 1989;83:1015–31.
14. Hofman, A., Ott, A., Breteler, M.M.B., Boots, M.L., Stooter, A.J.C., van Harskamp, F., van Druign, C.N., von Broeckhoven, C., and Arobbee, D.E. Atherosclerosis, apolipoprotein E, and prevalence of dementia and Alzheimer's disease in the Rotterdam Study. Lancet, Jan. 18, 1997;349:151–54.
15. Larkin, L., Moffett, R.J., and Teague, B. Regulation of apolipoprotein E production in macrophages. Int J Mol Med, 2000;6:253–58.
16. Roses, A.D. Apolipoprotein E and Alzheimer's disease. The tip of the susceptibility iceberg. Ann NY Acad Sci, Nov. 30, 1998;855:738–43.
17. Broscic, E., Bergerone, S., Gagnor, A., Colajanni, E., Matullo, G., Scaglione, L., Cassader, M., Gaschino, G., Di Leo, M., Brusca, A., Pagano, G.F., Piazza, A., and Trevi, G.P. Acute MI in young adults: prognostic role of apo E and other parameters at medium-term follow-up. Am Heart J, 2000;139:979–84.
18. Dzimiri, N., Meyer, B.F., Hussain, S.S., Basco, C., Afrane, B., and Halees, Z. Relevance of apo E polymorphism for CAD in the Saudi population, Arch Pathol and Lab Med, 1999;123:1241–45.
19. Kardia, S.L., Haviland, M.B., Ferrell, R.E., and Sing, C.F. The relationship between risk factor levels and presence of coronary artery calcification (CAC) is dependent on apo E genotype. Arterio Thromb and Vascular Biol, 1999;19:427–35.
20. Sparks, D.L. CAD, hypertension, apo E, and cholesterol: a link to Alzheimer's disease, Ann NY Acad Sci, 1997;826:128–46.
21. Brouwer, D.A., Jammison, P.T., and Cower, S.L. Clinical chemistry of common apoprotein E isoforms, J Chromatogr B Biomed Appl, 1996;678(1):23–41.
22. Weisgraber, K.H. Apolipoprotein E distribution among human plasma lipoproteins: role of the cysteine-arginine interchange at residue 112. J Lipid Res, 1990;31(8):1503–11.
23. Wu, M.L., Somjen, G.G., and Tombaugh, G.C. Mechanism of hydrogen peroxide and hydroxyl free radical-induced intracellular acidification in cultured rat cardiac myoblasts, Circ Res, 1996;78:564–72.
24. Smith, J.D. Apolipoprotein E4: an allele associated with many diseases. Ann Med, 2000;32:118–27.
25. Poirer, J., Davigno, J., Bouthillier, D., Kogan, S., Bertrand, P., and Gauthier, S. Lancet 342: 1993;697–9.
26. Saunders, A.M., Strittmatter, W.J., Schmechel, O., and St. George-Hyslop, P.H. Neurol 1993;43:1467–72.
27. Aw, T.Y., Jones, E., and Bates, T.J. Oral glutathione increases tissue glutathione in vivo, Chem Biol Interactions 1991;80:89–97.
28. Hunjan, M.K., and Evered, D.F. Absorption of glutathione from the gastrointestinal tract, Biochim Biophys Acta 1985;815:184–88.

15

Enriched Eggs for Human Consumption and the and Feeding Pattern of Layers

Carola García, Sergio Cornejo, and Cecilia Albala

Demographic and social changes have produced an increase in life expectancy and a shift in deaths from children to adults. Currently, the main causes of death are cardiovascular diseases, cancer, injuries, and congenital and metabolic conditions.[1] The high incidence of these diseases is related to malnutrition and sedentary and stressful lifestyles.[2] The rate of death attributable to ischemic heart disease has become the number one cause of adult death in the world, accounting for 7,200,000 deaths in 1997.[3]

As a consequence of urbanization, work becoming industrialized, and other factors, food habits have evolved to the consumption of highly refined, nutritionally concentrated products, increased levels of fat intake and saturated fatty acids, low intake of n-3 fatty acids, and other practices that hinder health. In developed countries, deaths due to ischemic heart disease have decreased from 51 percent in 1985 to 46 percent in 1997 due to a growing concern about the relationship between ischemic heart disease and nutrition, while in developing countries such deaths have increased from 16 to 24 percent, respectively.[3] All of these dietary practices are inherent to affluent, developed societies, which favor consumption of animal products (mainly red meats and milk products) that are a clear sign of "status."

When the United States is compared with east Asian Pacific developed societies like Japan, whose population lives under similar environmental and economic conditions, deaths from coronary heart disease in the United States and other developed Western countries exhibit a higher age adjusted rate (106.5/100,000 in the United States versus 30/100,000 in Japan, 1997).[4] Studies concerning dietary practices that can explain these epidemiological profiles in both societies show that the main sources of animal protein in typical east Asian diets are marine products like fish and seafood; terrestrial animals like cattle, pigs, and poultry provide animal protein (and fat) in the West.

In 1998, average per capita fish and seafood intakes were 66.5, 20.7, and 19.7 kg/year for Japan, the United States, and Europe, respectively; these figures have been virtually constant in Japan since 1978 and slightly higher in the United States and Europe. For the same period, meat per capita consumption in the United States has inceased from 106 to

122 kg/year, decreased from 76 to 72 kg/year in Europe, and increased from 28 to 42 kg/year in Japan.[5]

The reasons for the low fish and seafood consumption in Western societies are multicausal and lay in historical cultural patterns, reinforced by modern lifestyle; as such, these patterns are difficult to modify, at least in the short term.

As a consequence of the growing concern of consumers about risk factors for chronic diseases (including the cholesterol content of eggs and its possible adverse effects on health[6]), per capita egg consumption in the United States has decreased in the last decades: 290 to 235 eggs/year in 1970 and 1998, respectively. In the United Kingdom these figures were 275 and 225, respectively.[5] A similar trend has been observed in many other parts of the world, except for a few Asian and African countries whose intakes have been historically very low.

The avian industry is one of the most successful examples of the proper application of scientific and technological knowledge to improve the efficiency of animal production. Thirty years ago, under initial intensive industrial conditions of production, a broiler chicken took about 70 days to reach its market weight (1.4 and 1.8 kg for female and male chickens, respectively) with a feed conversion rate of 2.4 to 2.6 kg feed/kg live weight gain produced. Currently, it takes just 35 to 42 days and 1.8 to 1.9 kg feed for similar indexes of production. Similarly, eggs were produced with about 3.1 to 3.4 kg feed/kg egg and presently are produced with values ranging between 1.95 to 2.45; moreover, these products present better market and organoleptic characteristics, a greater diversity of alternatives for commercialization, relatively lower production costs per unit, and lower prices for consumers.

Eggs contain an almost ideal amino acid profile and significant levels of other nutrients like fat, vitamins, and minerals (Table 15.1); eggs can be produced under many management conditions ranging from simple domestic henhouses to highly industrialized laying enterprises that can lodge flocks of thousands of hens; eggs can be used in many culinary preparations and can be stored with just the common and ordinary precautions of refrigeration accorded to any fresh animal food, especially in relation to basic biosecurity rules. These characteristics make them an ideal source of nutrients, particularly for populations whose animal protein consumption is low because of the high prices of meat and milk products. Furthermore, it can be hypothesized that the phospholipids (PLs) that eggs contain may minimize the deleterious effects of cholesterol consumption. Moreover, the highly polyunsaturated fatty acid (PUFAs) esterified in those PLs are responsible for the decrease in the endogenous cholesterol synthesis under normal metabolic conditions.[7–9] In spite of this, nutritional and some genetic research efforts to decrease the cholesterol content of the egg have not been very successful, so we have to live with this characteristic inherent in a food of the highest biological value for the population.[10]

Fish, seafood, and their derivates exhibit a typical profile of fatty acids (FAs) in their fat: long-chain PUFAs of the n-3 series ranging from 18 to 22 atoms of carbon, mainly eicosapentanoic acid (EPA, C20:5 n-3), docosapentanoic acid (DPA, C22:5 n-3), and docosahexanoic acid (DHA, C22:6 n-3), comprise up to 30 percent of their fat's FAs; about 25 percent correspond to monounsaturated fatty acids (MUFAs), and the remaining

Table 15.1. Nutritional composition of yolk of large egg

Total weight	Energy	Water	Fat	Protein	Cholesterol
17 g	61 kcal	8.3 g	5.2 g	2.8 g	0.3 g

Fatty acids (weight and percentage of fat content)

Saturated	Monounsaturated	Polyunsaturated	Cholesterol
1.6 g (30.8)	2.0 g (38.5)	0.7 g (13.5)	218 mg

Minerals

Ca	P	Na	K	Mg	Fe	Zn	Cu	Mn
23 mg	83 mg	7 mg	16 mg	2 mg	0.6 mg	0.53 mg	0.004 mg	0.012 mg

Vitamins

A	C	B_1	B_2	Niacin	B_6	B_{12}	Folic acid	Pantothenic acid
331 IU	0	0.03 mg	0.11 mg	0	0.07 mg	0.53 mcg	25 mcg	0.65 mg

Source. Reference 14.

FAs are saturated (SFAs) (Table 15.2).[11–12] This profile gives their fats polyunsaturation indexes higher than those of other animal fats (0.9 to 1.5 versus 0.04 for lamb fat to 0.7 for the fat of chickens fed corn-based diets) and makes them foodstuffs with unique functional and nutritional properties.[13] Fish oils and fish meal lipids have high digestibilities and energy values in all animals tested and have been proved very succesful ingredients for enhancing growth and production indexes in all types of farm animals.[12] Some vegetable oils, like flaxseed oil, cottonseed oil, sunflower oil, canola oil, and others, exhibit very high polyunsaturation indexes and also contain n-3 FAs,[14] but in a lesser quantity than the marine lipids (Table 15.3).

PUFAs are essential nutrients. They are important components of cellular membranes and exert outstanding roles in many biological functions, as in the platelet aggregation mechanisms, the function of receptors of neurotransmitters and insulin, and the immune system of all known animals. n-3 FAs and their relationship with n-6 FAs have been extensively studied in avian experiments. Almost all of the studies concluded that these nutrients exert a beneficial influence upon the humoral and cellular immunity of the birds by different mechanisms: in some cases decreasing the cytotoxicity of some eicosanoids normally produced, in other cases increasing the mitotic rate of specialized cell populations related to the production of specific antibodies, and in many cases modulating the balance of enzyme pathways that control prostaglandins, tromboxanes, and leukotrienes.[15–18]

All the functions listed here depend on the proper relationship between the n-6 and n-3 series of FAs, as well as their chain length.[19] It is estimated that a balanced diet with respect to the supply of n-6:n-3 FAs must present a ratio of 4:1 to 5:1. Relationships of higher magnitude may imply a serious deficiency of the long-chain PUFAs of the n-3 series. Metabolically, the biochemical transformations within the three families of FAs

Table 15.2. Iodine values, weight percentage of saturated fatty acids, monounsaturated fatty acids and EPA + DHA of some major marine oils

		Iodine values	SFA (%)	MUFA (%) C20:1 + C22:1)	PUFA (%) (EPA + DHA)
Body oils	Herring (Atlantic)	125	19	35	14
	Capelin	125	18	36	11
	Redfish	125	21	36	9
	Herring (Pacific)	140	34	10	7
	Sand launce	140	24	27	17
	Mackerel	150	27	38	15
	Salmon (Pacific)	150	36	17	19
	Sardine	160	30	8	24
	Menhaden	162	32	2	20
	Anchovy	181	30	3	26
	Pilchard	185	28	5	26
Liver oils	Cod (Atlantic)	165	21	13	24
	Pollock (Alaska)	160	18	30	17
	Squid (Pacific)	180	21	17	28
Other	Salmon egg (Pacific)	210	¿?	¿?	38
	Seal (Atlantic)	150	14	17	14

Source. References 11 and 12.
Note. SFA = saturated fatty acid; MUFA = monounsaturated fatty acid; PUFA = polyunsaturated fatty acid; EPA = eicosapentanoic acid; DHA = docosahexanoic acid.

Table 15.3. Composition of some fish and vegetable oils (%)

	SFA (%)	MUFA (%)	PUFA (%)	PUFA:SFA
Herring oil	21.4	56.4	15.7	0.73
Menhaden oil (hydrogenated)	88.6	0.0	0.0	—
Salmon oil	14.3	29.3	40.0	2.790
Sardine oil	30.0	33.6	32.1	1.070
Canola oil	7.1	58.6	29.3	41.300
Coconut oil	86.4	5.7	2.1	0.024
Corn oil	12.9	24.3	58.6	4.540
Cottonseed oil	25.7	17.9	52.1	2.030
Olive oil	13.6	73.6	8.6	0.630
Palm kernel oil	6.9	5.2	1.3	0.190
Peanut oil	17.7	46.4	32.1	1.810
Safflower oil	9.3	12.1	74.3	7.990
Soybean oil	15.0	42.9	37.9	2.530
Sunflower oil	10.0	19.3	65.7	6.570

Source. Reference 14.
Note. SFA = saturated fatty acid; MUFA = monounsaturated fatty acid; PUFA = polyunsaturated fatty acid.

(n-3, n-6, and n-9) depend on the mutual competition that these FAs exert upon the Δ-6 and Δ-5 desaturase enzymes, resulting in the importance of an appropriate relationship between the FA series in the fats and oils consumed.[20]

Marine fats and oils, due to their long-chain PUFA content, have important cardio-protective effects by being able to lower low-density lipoprotein (LDL) cholesterol, promote vasodilation, and inhibit platelet aggregation.[21] This association was virtually demonstrated when the relation of eskimo diets (high in marine FAs) and low rates of cardiovascular diseases was reported.[22]

As already discussed, many people in Western societies are reluctant to increase their consumption of fish and other marine products and prefer those foods that contain terrestrial animal meat, eggs, and refined carbohydrates. Consequently, an interesting strategy has been developed in the last 20 years: those "desired" foodstuffs have been enriched with "desirable" nutrients to increase the consumption of the nutrients without altering deeply rooted food habits that, despite the efforts that have already been made, will not be modified without much more education.

The products of nonruminant species (meat, eggs, and milk) very closely reflect their feeding pattern of fat and amino acids. This condition is a useful tool for the development of the following strategy: if nonruminant species are fed "desirable" nutrients, the "desired" products can be obtained for human use.

Nutrition can influence many of the quality characteristics of eggs, such as their size and the proportion of their main constituents: yolk and albumen. Dietary changes have little effect on the overall composition of albumen and yolk in terms of dry matter content and amino acid composition; however, micronutrient and FA composition can be modified.[23]

Recently, these changes have taken a new significance in relation to human health, particularly in the area of n-3 FAs,[23] and the modification of the lipid profile of egg yolk by dietary manipulations has been studied by many authors that have established that enriched eggs would be a source of FAs with beneficial health effects;[24–30] currently, there are market eggs enriched with n-3 FAs—both from marine and vegetable sources—in Europe, the United States, and South America, mainly in Brazil and Chile.

Corn, milo, barley, and oats are the major coarse grains used for feeding poultry, mainly for energy supply in the diets. Occasionally surplus or frost-damaged wheat is sufficiently low priced to compete with the coarse cereals used for poultry feeds. In some areas of the world, broken rice is a low-cost energy source. Some cereal byproducts like those resulting from dry and wet milling of corn (hominy feed, corn bran, corn germ cake, and corn germ meal), those from the milling process of wheat (wheat bran, wheat middlings, wheat shorts, etc.), and screenings (the residual material obtained in the process of cleaning grain and seeds) are also used in hens' diets.

Soybean meal, corn gluten meal, cottonseed meal, and peanut meal represent the major plant protein supplements used in poultry feeds. Other plant protein supplements used in hens' diets are decorticated safflower seed meal, sesame meal, sunflower seed meal, rapeseed meal, linseed meal, and coconut oil meal.

Protein sources derived from animal products have been prized for many years for animal feeding. Fish meal, meat meal, and tankage and poultry industry byproducts have been used in hen diets.

The most concentrated sources of energy used in poultry feeding are fats and oils that are available from the meat-processing industry, from byproducts of the manufacture of soaps and refining of vegetable oils, or vegetable or fish oils themselves. For a long time these materials were included in hen diets only for energetic purposes because of their high energy concentration and the desirable qualities that they add to feeds (less dustiness and improved palatability). Because there is more concern about the quality of fats, their fatty acid composition, and the beneficial effects that they can transfer to other animal products, they must be defined to enable prediction of the nutritional value of any particular product.

Some products resulting from fermentation of various grains have been used in poultry diets; examples of these products are dried or irradiated yeasts from the brewing or distilling industry. Other byproducts, such as molasses, result from the sugar industry based on cane or beet; they are a cheap source of carbohydrates and can be used in up to 4–5 percent of diets because of their high mineral content.

Research to modify the lipid profile of yolk fat has been focused on the utilization of both vegetable and marine souces of FAs, the single n-3 FA, and, to a lesser extent, marine algae. Such modifications, directed essentially to increasing n-3 FAs, began with the incorporation of fish oils and meals. The frequent appearance of undesirable organoleptic characters led to the development of alternative diet integration approaches (utilizing, for example, marine algae–based feed integrations and microencapsulation) and to the reconsideration of the use of plant α-linolenic acid (α-LNA, C:3, n-3) sources such as flax, colza, and soy in layers' feeding.

The production of eggs requires the deposition of large amounts of yolk lipids, mostly during the days prior to ovulation. Yolk lipids and proteins are synthesized in the liver under the influence of estrogen and progesterone and are transferred through the blood to the ovarian follicles. Lipids in the yolk are of two main types: lipoproteins (LPs) and vitellogenins (VGs). In the chicken, LPs contribute about 95 percent of the yolk lipids. The liver packages and secretes triglycerides (TGs) and phospholipids (PLs) in a special yolk-targeted VLDL (VLDLy), which has unique structural and biochemical properties for targeting it to the ovary. VLDLy is half the size of normal VLDL and has apolipoprotein VLDL II on its surface, making it a poor substrate for lipoprotein lipase. Consequently, the TGs in VLDLy are not well used by skeletal muscle or adipose tissue. Its small size permits it to pass through the granulosa basal lamina of the ovarian follicle and bind to the apolipoprotein B receptor of the oolemma. It is endocytosed intact to form the yolk. The sievinglike action of the ovarian-follicle basal lamina prevents the uptake of portomicrons arriving from the diet. This combination of follicular ultrastructure and VLDLy size allows dietary fat to be modified by the liver prior to inclusion into the yolk of eggs, permitting better control of yolk lipid characteristics by the female.[18] This hepatic modification is not complete, however, and yolk lipid composition still reflects that of the diet, especially in content of PUFAs.[31]

Hargis et al.[30] studied the effect of a standard laying hen diet enriched with 3 percent menhaden oil, versus an isocaloric control diet with no added fat, on the lipid profile of shell egg yolk. Menhaden oil did not affect any productive parameter, total yolk fat, or yolk cholesterol contents. However, yolk contents of n-6 and n-3 FAs were influenced by the diet. Arachidonic acid (AA, C20:4, n-6) decreased and eicosapentanoic acid (EPA) increased after 1 week with the menhaden diet, and 1 and 2 weeks later linoleic acid (LA, C:18:2, n-6) and DHA acid increased respectively. These changes resulted in a decrease in the ratio of n-6 to n-3 FAs from 18 to 3 for eggs from hens fed the control and experimental diets respectively.

García and Albala[32] analyzed eggs from hens fed marine (fish meal) and vegetable (soy meal) sources of FAs. Their results showed that eggs from hens fed marine products, an ordinary practice in Chile where fish meal is relatively cheap and is used on average in 3–4 percent of layers' diets, contain significantly less cholesterol (0.92 versus 1.29 g/100 g yolk) and fewer TGs and PLs than those of hens fed only vegetable feeds. Even though there were no significant differences in the total proportions of SFAs, MUFAs, and PUFAs in the yolk, n-3 FAs—mainly EPA and DHA—were significantly higher (1.7 and 4 times, respectively) and n-6 were 30 percent lower in the eggs of hens fed marine products (Table 15.4).

Grashorn and Steinhilber[33] studied the effect of different n-6:n-3 relations in the diets of hens. These relations were obtained by means of the addition of fats with different fatty acid compositions to a basal diet to make a diet with 17 percent crude protein and 11.6 MJ metabolizable energy/kg. The fats used were mixtures of soybean oil, linseed oil, rapeseed oil, sunflower oil and /or fish oil at a level of fat addition of 2.5 percent. The n-6:n-3 relations studied were 10:1, 5:1, 3:1, 1:1, 1:3, and 1:5. In the yolks the percentage of total n-3 FAs increased with increasing levels of n-3 in the diets, and the relation between n-6 and n-3 decreased, corresponding quite well to the relations in the diets. Nevertheless, it seems to be hardly possible to increase n-3 FAs over the proportion 3:1 because there may exist a threshold for the accumulation of n-3 in the yolks. This may be due to the relation between LA and α-LA in the diets used. Even in the diet with the highest amount of n-3 FAs, the proportion of LA is higher by the factor 1.5 than the proportion of α-LA. This

Table 15.4. Lipid profile of egg yolk and its relation to the feeding pattern of hens

Fatty acids in yolk lipids (g/100 g)	Feeding pattern of hens based on: Marine products	Vegetable products
Saturated	43.26 ± 1.11	43.80 ± 2.15
Monounsaturated	31.67 ± 2.13	32.23 ± 1.08
Polyunsaturated	23.07 ± 1.82	22.98 ± 2.88
Total n-3	7.13 ± 0.83[a]	1.77 ± 0.55[b]
C20:5 n-3 (EPA)	0.57 ± 0.25[a]	0.33 ± 0.02[b]
C22:6 n-3 (DHA)	5.96 ± 0.59[a]	1.40 ± 0.44[b]
Total n-6	15.71 ± 2.51[a]	20.88 ± 2.32[b]

Source. Reference 32.
Note. EPA = eicosapentanoic acid; DHA = docosahexanoic acid.
[a]Significantly different from saturated ($P < 0.05$).
[b]Significantly different from marine product fed ($P < 0.05$).

means the n-6 pathway is favored in the metabolism of the hen, limiting the transformation of LA to EPA and DHA. Therefore, the proportion of LA is 4.4 times higher in yolks than the proportion of α-LA. In general, the use of linseed oil in the diet will result in higher proportions of n-3 FAs in the yolks than the use of fish oil due to linseed oil's higher content of n-3 FAs. TBAR values were very low, so the oxidative processes may still be of no importance; probably the content of α-tocopherol in the yolk was high enough to compensate for oxidative processes. These authors suggested that a distinct enrichment of eggs with EPA and DHA and/or other n-3 FAs may only be achieved by using pure FAs instead of oils.

Other authors have used mixtures of cereals varying in their FA composition to modify the yolk lipid profile; Kaminska,[34] used different mixtures of maize, barley, dehulled oats, wheat, and fish meal. These mixtures had varying levels of LA. Including 20–40 percent dehulled oats in the diet decreased the content of MUFAs and elevated the content of PUFAs. Eggs from hens fed diets in which maize was fortified with 20–40 percent of dehulled oats contained more LA than eggs from hens fed other diets. The increased content of LA acompanying an increased proportion of dietary oats was reported previously by other authors.[35] Feeding oats, especially barley, caused a highly significant increase in α-LA and DHA compared with maize. The highest level of DHA was found when a barley-wheat diet was supplemented with 2 percent fish meal. The addition of fish meal decreased PUFA n-6 and increased PUFA n-3. Inclusion of 30 percent barley in the diet caused the n-6:n-3 ratio to decrease very significantly. This ratio (5.11:1) is close to the ideal ratio suggested by Sincler, quoted by Farrell.[36] The narrowest ratio (4.69:1) was achieved after supplementing the barley-wheat diet with fish meal.

Evans et al.[37] studied the effect of the addition of a vegetable source of fat by means of 2.5 percent cottonseed oil to the diet of laying hens; their results showed that there were no changes in yolk VLDL and LDL and the fatty acid composition of those lipid fractions did not differ from those of the control group. Lipids of all the different LPs isolated from egg yolk contained more stearic and less oleic and palmitoleic acids than did those of control hens. The increased content of stearic acid increased the density of the lipoproteins so that a larger proportion of the LPs were in the LDL and a smaller portion in the VLDL fractions of yolk lipids.

The effect of the addition of saturated and unsaturated FAs and cholesterol to the diet of laying hens was studied by Sim and Bragg.[38] The sources of fat used were 8 percent hydrogenated coconut oil or safflower oil with or without either cholesterol or soysterols or both. Both cholesterol and soysterol decreased oleic acid and decreased palmitic and/or stearic acid of the yolk. These changes were significantly greater upon feeding of cholesterol than soysterol. However, when both sterols were added simultaneously, the effect decreased greatly.

Mixtures of steam-pelleted barley and full-fat canola seed at different proportions (80:20; 70:30; 60:40; 50:50) in pullet diets were evaluated.[39] These mixtures were used at the 40 percent dietary level in isonitrogenous, isocaloric diets. Yolk color index and contents of LA, α-LA, and DHA increased linearly as full-fat canola seed content of the diets increased, suggesting that this source of n-3 FAs may provide an alternative for the enrichment of shell eggs with these healthful nutrient components.

Results by Ferrier et al.[29] showed that feeding diets containing 0, 10, or 20 percent flaxseed to Leghorn pullets provided a marked progressive increase in n-3 yolk FAs. The n-3 acids were α-LA (28, 261, and 527 mg/egg, respectively) and DHA (51, 81, and 87 mg/egg, respectively). These authors, after a clinical trial with male volunteers, reported that the inclusion of flaxseed in the diets of laying hens, and its correlate in the eggs produced, represents an important nutritional source of n-3 FAs.

Jiang et al.[40] fed hens diets high in oleic acid (OA, C18:1, n-9), α-LA, or LA prepared by incorporation of high-oleic sunflower seed, full-fat flax seed, or regular high-LA sunflower seed, respectively, to study the effects of dietary fats on the FA profile of major lipid classes of poultry eggs. After 3 weeks of feeding, the FA composition of yolk total lipids, TGs, phosphatidylcholine (PC), and phosphatidylethanolamine (PE) were measured by gas chromatography. Dietary treatments had no effects on yolk total lipid content. Feeding high-OA sunflower seed increased yolk OA by 17 percent, and this change affected only the TGs. The increases of yolk LA and AA upon high-LA sunflower seed were distributed evenly among TGs and PC with moderate effect on the PE fraction. The enrichment of LA in eggs from the flax regime was mainly in TGs. The longer-chain FAs, such as EPA, DPA, and DHA, were deposited exclusively in PLs, particularly in PE. The contents of the longer-chain n-3 FAs in PE were three to seven times those in PC, indicating a preferential incorporation in that phospholipid fraction.

Ground and whole flaxseed at levels of 5 or 15 percent were used by Aymond[41] to enrich egg yolk fat with n-3 FAs; the author compared the lipid profile and yolk oxidation quality with those of eggs enriched by means of 1.5 percent menhaden oil. All the treatments increased n-3 FA content in the yolk (α-LA, EPA, and DHA for flaxseed and EPA and DHA for menhaden oil), but at the 15 percent flaxseed level, the increase in n-3 FAs was higher when the seed was ground than when the whole seed was used. The oxidative quality of the yolk lipids wasn't affected by the incorporation of the n-3 saturated FAs as reflected by the determination of TBAR.

Collins[42] investigated whether pearl millet, when substituted for corn in laying hen diets, would enrich egg yolks with n-3 FAs. Diets were isoenergetic and isocalorically formulated with corn, equal amounts of corn and pearl millet, and pearl millet as grain sources. The substitution of pearl millet for corn decreased the ratio of n-6 to n-3 FAs (13.1:1; 10.1:1; and 8.3:1 respectively), showing clearly that pearl millet inclusion produces eggs significantly enriched in n-3 FAs.

In another study, the addition of 3 percent α-LA to the diet of hens increased the amount of n-3 FAs of the yolk by 6.5 percent—70 percent as α-LA, 20 to 25 percent as DHA, and the remaining 5 to 10 percent as DPA.[43]

Some authors have studied the supplementation of hen diets with α-tocopherol in order to prevent oxidation of unsatutated FAs when these FAs are increased to enrich eggs. These authors reported that the content of α-tocopherol in eggs increases in a dose-dependent manner.[44–46] Galobart et al.[47] studied the effect of the addition of increasing levels of α-tocopheryl acetate to a basal diet containing 5 percent linseed oil (65 percent PUFAs, 34.3 percent n-3) and how it affects storage stability. Their results showed that the vitamin E content of eggs decreases with processing and storage time; thus, the level required in hens' diets should be adjusted depending not only on the fatty acid composition of the eggs but also on the conditions of processing and conditions and time of storage.

These same authors[48] investigated the effect of vitamin E and canthaxanthin and their relation with n-3 or n-6 FA supplementation. They found that n-3 FA–enriched eggs are more susceptible to oxidation than those enriched with n-6 FAs and that the addition of 200 ppm of vitamin E reduces the oxidation induced by the spray-drying process, but supplementation with 5 ppm of canthaxanthin had no significant effect as an antioxidant.

The enrichment of eggs with a vegetable fatty acid blend, linseed oil, and fish oil supplemented with crushed and spray-dried aplanospores of the green micro alga *Hematococcus pluvialis* to provide 0.2 or 4 mg of astaxanthin per kg feed was studied by Elwinger and Inborr.[49] The deposition rates of carotenoids and astaxanthin in the egg yolk were 14 and 10 percent, respectively. Peroxide values of the feed containing linseed oil without added algal meal tended to be elevated, whereas addition of algal meal to the diets decreased the peroxide value. The anisidine value of egg yolks followed the same pattern, indicating antioxidant activity of the algal meal. The content of n-3 FAs was highest in eggs from hens fed linseed oil. The content of EPA plus DHA was calculated to be 223, 106, and 85 mg per egg in eggs from hens fed fish oil, linseed oil, and vegetable fatty acid blend, respectively. Stored eggs from hens fed fish oil were categorized as having a "stronger egg taste" by a taste panel. Otherwise there were no remarkable gastronomic differences, either in fresh or in stored eggs, due to fat or astaxanthin supplementation.

An experiment carried out by Mozzon et al.[50] was aimed at the evaluation of the efficiency of the transfer of n-3 PUFAs (EPA and DHA) to the eggs of hens given diets integrated with these components. The integrators utilized were made up of an appropriate mixture of fats from different sources, supplied as microspheres obtained through a technology analogous to spray-drying. Fish oils represented the source of n-3 FAs: their mixing with silica and fractionated palm oil appeared to allow a proportional decrease in the microsphere structure of the surface-exposed PUFAs. This, together with the addition of appropriate concentrations of tocopherols, allowed sufficient antioxidant protection of PUFAs, preventing oxidation and consequently preventing health problems and the appearance of negative organoleptic characters in the final product. The total amount of PUFAs in the eggs was higher than that of a control group. Regarding the individual PUFA content, enriched eggs containing EPA—not present in control nonenriched eggs—had higher content of DHA and DPA and lower content of AA.

The "enrichment" strategy already commented on, with marine oils or meals, overcomes the "fishy" taste or smell transmitted to the enriched products. This condition has been evaluated in different experiments carried out by submitting the different avian products obtained (eggs and meats) to sensorial evaluations made by trained panels of experts. In general, when the marine sources of lipids did not exceed 5–8 percent of the diets, the different panelists could not distinguish between egg types.[9,51–52]

Fish taste doesn't seem to be a problem when fish FAs are used to enrich eggs, providing that all the technological processes involved in the production of marine meals and oils have been adequately controlled and that the eggs are conveniently stored and commercialized within a reasonable time. When other sources of FAs are used, mainly from vegetable oil seeds, this "fishy taste" problem is absent.

Dried-fermented algae can contain over 7 percent DHA in naturally encapsulated form. Herber[53] investigated the use of a natural golden marine algae in laying hen diets to incorporate n-3 FAs into yolk lipids. This algae is unique in its FA profile due to its high content of DHA and the absence of other n-3 FAs normally present in marine oils such as menhaden oil. In two experiments, conducted with different levels of incorporation of the algae and menhaden oil (compared with the typical corn-soybean diets fed to hens), the supplementation with marine products significantly increased yolk total n-3 FAs with concomitant reductions in yolk n-6 FAs. Although menhaden oil diets contained predominantly EPA, the main FA deposited was DHA. Marine algae also promoted an efficient deposition of DHA, the highest concentrations being attained when it was fed at 4.8 percent of the diet (180 mg total n-3 FAs). This data indicates that the use of this algae as a direct source of dietary n-3 FAs may be an efficient alternative to current sources of n-3 FAs for the supplementation of poultry diets for the enrichment of eggs.

Herber and Van Elswyk[54] utilized a microalgal product enriched with DHA as a source of n-3 FAs. The diets were supplemented at the 2.4 or 4.8 percent level. The results showed that the n-3 FA content of yolk lipids increased with the supplementation and that consumer acceptability of the eggs remained unaffected by the enrichment with n-3 FAs.

These marine algal products provide perhaps one of the most effective ways of producing n-3–enriched eggs.

The use of some crustaceans (*Mexican langostilla*) as meals in the diets of white layer hens was reported to provide an excellent way to incorporate adequate amounts—and proper proportions—of n-3 and n-6 FAs into eggs, without any adverse effect on the productivity of the hens.[55]

The effect of supplementation of hen diets with different products to decrease the cholesterol content of shell eggs has been studied. Beyer and Jensen[56] studied the effect of orotic acid in the diet on the cholesterol content of eggs. There were no effects from its addition on egg weight, yolk weight, percentage of yolk, or egg production. However, the data indicated that orotic acid is ineffective for reducing egg cholesterol levels.

The effect of supplemental niacin on laying hen performance and egg cholesterol content was investigated by Leeson et al.[57] Dietary niacin level had no effect on cholesterol content of eggs, even when levels as high as 1.022 mg/kg, which closely simulates therapeutic levels used for humans, were added.

Beyer and Jensen[58] used α-ketoisocaproic acid and leucine in laying hen diets to test whether these substances at different levels could modify egg cholesterol and layer performance. They found that 0.09 percent α-ketoisocaproic acid and 0.09 percent leucine significantly reduced egg cholesterol after 4 weeks' intervention. After 8 weeks 0.27 percent α-ketoisocaproic reduced egg cholesterol significantly below controls.

Cholesterol content of eggs is difficult to manipulate by nutrition or other genetic or pharmacological methods; it has been suggested that the hen will cease laying when egg cholesterol content is lowered below the amount necessary to sustain embryonic development.[59] Clinical studies with normolipaemic individuals showed that they can eat two eggs per day[60–61] or up to four n-3–enriched eggs per day[62] as part of a moderate fat diet not exceeding 30 percent of calories from fat and 10 percent as SFAs without alteration in their lipid profiles.

Finally, it appears very clear that the nutritional enrichment of eggs is not only possible but necessary. This can be done in different ways depending on the local availability of foodstuffs and their costs. In the southern Pacific hemisphere, fish products are probably the most adequate source of n-3 FAs because they are normally available at convenient prices, whereas in other parts of the world, especially on the Atlantic coast of South America and in the northern hemisphere, cereals, oil seeds, and algae are the best resources. In the near future structured lipids with a desired chemical configuration will be widely available, and their incorporation in layer diets will most likely represent the most adequate way to enrich eggs and other foodstuffs with specific FAs.

Another fact that must be taken into account when deciding the best strategy for enrichment of eggs is the additional benefit in the birds that the egg producers have when using appropriate n-3:n-6 ratios in the layers' diets. It has already been proven that they will improve the cellular as well as the humoral immune responses of the birds. This sanitary "plus" must be taken into account when comparing the economic profit of the enrichment strategy with the direct costs of the enrichment.

Eggs have been stigmatized because of their cholesterol content; this has masked their nutritional advantages: quality protein, vitamin and mineral supplies, energetic content, and, in the case of enriched eggs, lipid profile. According to the American Dietary Guidelines,[63] healthy people can eat up to 300 mg/day of cholesterol, so when their diets are adjusted to these nutrient recommendations, eating three to four eggs per week won't be dangerous at all; moreover, if eggs are higher in n-3 FAs and the proportion of SFAs recommended is not exceeded, they can represent a source of beneficial nutrients.

The price of enriched shell eggs will depend on the source of FAs incorporated and the technological processes needed for modification. Their cost and consumer concerns about their benefits will determine the convenience and feasibility of their production.

The enrichment of eggs may increase their market price, but once consumers are aware of their health benefits, they should be well disposed to spend more to obtain their extra advantages.

References

1. Albala, C., and Vio, F. Epidemiological transition in Latin America: the case of Chile. Public Health 1995;109:431–42.
2. Multiple Risk Factor Intervention Trial Research Group. Risk factor changes and mortality results. Am Med Assoc 1982;248:1465–77.
3. Organisation Mondiale de la Santé. Rapport sur la Santé dans le Monde. Genève. La vie au 21 siècle. Une perspective pour tous. Rapport du Directeur Général, 1998.
4. World Health Organization. World Health Statistics Annual. 1997–1999. http://www.who.int/.
5. Food Agriculture Organization. United Nations. Food Balance Sheets. 2000. http://www.fao.org/.

6. Brown, D.J., and Schrader, L.F. Cholesterol information and shell egg consumption. Am J Agric Econ 1990;72:548–55.
7. Hargis, P.S. Modifying egg yolk cholesterol in the domestic fowl: a review. World's Poult Sci J 1988;44:17–29.
8. Oh, S.Y., Lin, C.H., Ryue, J., and Bell, D.E. Eggs enriched with omega-3 fatty acids as a wholesome food. J Appl Nutr 1994;46(1–2):14–25.
9. Leskanich, C.O., and Noble, R.C. Manipulation of n-3 polyunsaturated fatty acid composition of avian eggs and meat. World's Poult Sci Assoc 1998;53:155–83.
10. Whitehead, C.C. Nutrition and egg quality. In Eggs and Eggs Products Quality. Proceedings of VIII European Symposium on the Quality of Eggs and Egg Products, vol. II. Bologna, Italy, Sept. 19–23, 1999.
11. Ackman, R. The year of the fish oils. Oils and fats group international lecture. Chem Ind, Mar. 7, 1988.
12. Opstvedt, J. Fish lipids in animal nutrition. International Association of Fish Meal Manufacturers. IAFMM, N[er] 1985;22:1–27.
13. Stolpher, Bloch A., and Shils, M.E. Nutrition Facts Manual: A Quick Reference. Baltimore: Williams and Wilkins, 1996, pp. 137–42.
14. Bowes, Anna de Planter. Bowes and Church's Food Values of Portions Commonly Used. 17th ed. Philadelphia, New York:Lippincott, 1998.
15. Cook, M.E., Miller, C.C., Park, Y., and Pariza, M. Immune modulation by altered nutrient metabolism: nutritional control of immune-induced growth depression. Poult Sci 1993;72:1301—5.
16. Cherian, G., and Sim, J.S. Net transfer and incorporation of yolk n-3 fatty acids into developing chick embryos. Poult Sci 1993;72:98–105.
17. Fritsche, K., and Cassity, N. Dietary n-3 fatty acids reduce antibody-dependent cell cytotoxicity and alter eicosanoid release by chicken immune cells. Poult Sci 1992;71:1646–57.
18. Klasing, K.C. Lipids. In Comparative Avian Nutrition, chap. 7. Wallingford, UK: CAB International, University Press, 1998, pp 171–200.
19. Valenzuela, A., Sanhuesa, J., and y Garrido A. Acidos grasos poliinsaturados de cadena larga n-3: cuándo y porqué es necesaria la suplementación con estos ácidos grasos. Aceites y grasas. Junio 1999:294–99.
20. Valenzuela, A., and y Garrido, A. Importancia nutricional de los ácidos grasos poliinsaturados n-3 de cadena larga : el beneficio de su suplementación. Rev Chil Nutr 1998;25(3):21–29.
21. Uauy, R., and Valenzuela, A. Marine oils as a source of omega-3 fatty acids in the diet: how to optimize the health benefits. Prog Food Nutr Sci 1992;16:199–243.
22. Dyerberg, J., Bang, H.O., Stoffersen, E., Moncada, S., and Vane, J.R. Eicosapentanoic acid and prevention of thrombosis and atherosclerosis? Lancet 1978;2(8081):117–19.
23. Whitehead, C.C. Nutrition and egg quality. In Eggs and Eggs Products Quality, Proceedings of VIII European Symposium on the Quality of Eggs and Egg Products, vol. II. Bologna, Italy, Sept. 19–23, 1999.
24. Edington, J., Geekie, M., Carter, R., Benfield, L., Fisher, K., Ball, M., and Mann, J. Effect of dietary cholesterol on plasma cholesterol concentration in subjects following reduced fat, high fibre diet. Br Med J Clin Res Ed, Feb. 7, 1987;294(6568):333–36.
25. Edington, J., Geekie, M., Carter, R., Benfield, L., Ball, M., and Mann, J. Serum lipid response to dietary cholesterol in subjects fed a low fat, high fibre diet. Am J Clin Nutr 1989;50(1):58–62.
26. Oh, Sy, Ryue, J., Hsieh, C.H., and Bell, D.E. Eggs enriched in omega-3 fatty acids and alterations in lipid concentrations in plasma and lipoproteins and blood pressure. Am J Clin Nutr 1991;54(4):689–95.

27. Garwin, J.L., Morgan, J.M., Stowell, R.L., Richardson, M.P., Walker, M.C., and Capuzzi, D.M. Modified eggs are compatible with a diet that reduces serum cholesterol concentration in humans. J Nutr 1992;122:2153–216.
28. Jiang, Z., and Sim, J.S. Consumption of n-3 polyunsaturated fatty acid-enriched eggs and changes in plasma lipids of human subjects. Nutrition 1993;9(6):513–18.
29. Ferrier, L.K., Caston, L.J., Leeson, S., Squires, J., Weaver, B.J., and Holub, B.J. Alpha linolenic and docosahexanoic acid enriched eggs from hens fed flaxseed; influence on blood lipids and platelet phospholipid fatty acids in humans. Am J Clin Nutr 1995;62(1):81–86.
30. Hargis, P.S., Van Elswyk, M.E., and Hargis, B.M. Dietary modification of yolk lipid with menhaden oil. Poult Sci 1991;70(4):874–83.
31. Noble, R.C., Speake, B.K., Mc Cartney, R., Foggin, C.M., and Deeming, D.C. Yolk lipids and their fatty acids in the wild and captive ostrich (*Strutio camelus*). Comp Biochem Physiol–Biochem and Molec Biol 1996;113:753–56.
32. García, C., and Albala, C. Composición lipídica de huevos de gallinas alimentadas con productos grasos y proteicos marinos. Arch Lat Nutr 1998;48(1):71–76.
33. Grashorn, M.A., and Steinhilber, S. Effect of dietary fat with different relations between omega-6 and omega-3 fatty acids on egg quality. In Eggs and Eggs Products Quality, Proceedings of VIII European Symposium on the Quality of Eggs and Egg Products, vol. II. Bologna, Italy, Sept. 19–23, 1999.
34. Kaminska, B.Z. Fatty acid profiles of egg yolks as influenced by diets containing high levels of maize, dehulled oats or barley and fish meal supplement. In Eggs and Eggs Products Quality, Proceedings of VIII European Symposium on the Quality of Eggs and Egg Products, vol. II. Bologna, Italy, Sept. 19–23,1999.
35. Aimonen, E.M.J., and Uusi-Rauva, E. Replacement of barley by oats and enzyme supplementation in diets from laying hens. 2. Interior quality and chemical composition of eggs. Acta Agric Scand 1991;41:193–205.
36. Farrell, D.J. The problems and practicalities of producing an omega-3 fortified egg. In Eggs and Eggs Products Quality, Proceedings of VI European Symposium on the Quality of Eggs and Egg Products. Zaragoza, Sept. 25–29, 1995, pp. 351–60.
37. Evans, R.J., Flegal, C.J., Foerder, C.A., Bauer, D.H., and La Vigne, M. The influence of crude cottonseed oil in the feed on the blood and egg lipoproteins of laying hens. Poult Sci 1997;56(2):268–79.
38. Sim, J.S., and Bragg, D.B. Effect of dietary oil, cholesterol and soysterols on the lipid concentration and fatty acid composition of egg yolk, liver and serum of laying hens. Poult Sci 1978;57(2):466–72.
39. Nwokolo, E., and Sim, J. Barley and full-fat canola seed in layer diets. Poult Sci 1989;68(11):1485–89.
40. Jiang, Z.R., Ahn, D.U., and Sim, J.S. Effects of feeding flax and two types of sunflower seeds on fatty acid compositions of yolk lipid classes. Poult Sci 1991;70(12):2467–75.
41. Aymond, W.M. Yolk thiobarbituric acid reactive substances and n-3 fatty acids in response to whole and ground flaxseed. Poult Sci 1995;74(8):1388–94.
42. Collins, V.P. Pearl millet in layer hen diets enhances egg yolk n-3 fatty acids. Poult Sci 1997;76(2):326–30.
43. Ahn, D.U., Sunwoo, H.H., Wolfe, F.H., and Sim J.S. Effects of dietary alpha linolenic acid and strain of hen on the fatty acid composition, storage stability and flavor characteristics of chicken eggs. Poult Sci 1995;74(9):1540–47.
44. Whale, K.W.J., Hoppe, P.P., and McIntosh, G. Effects of storage and various intrinsic vitamin

E concentrations on lipid oxidation in dried egg powders. J Sci Food Agric 1993;61:463–69.

45. Jiang, Y.H., Ma Geachin, R.B., and Bailey, C.A. α tocopherol, β carotene and retinol enrichment of chicken eggs. Poult Sci 1994;73:1137–43.
46. Surai, P.F., Ionov, L.A., Kuklenko, T.V., Kostjuk, I.A., and Mac Pherson, A. Effect of supplementing the hen's diet with vitamin A on the accumulation of vitamins A and E, ascorbic acid and carotenoids in the egg yolk and in the embryonic liver. Br Poult Sci 1998;39:257–63.
47. Galobart, J., Barroeta, A.C., Baucells, M.D., and Guardiola, F. Vitamin E levels and lipid oxidation in n-3 fatty acids enriched eggs. In Eggs and Eggs Products Quality, Proceedings of VIII European Symposium on the Quality of Eggs and Egg Products, vol. II. Bologna, Italy, Sept. 19–23, 1999.
48. Galobart, J., Barroeta, A.C., Baucells, M.D., and Guardiola, F. 1999. Oxidation in fresh and spray-dried n-3 and n-6 fatty acid enriched eggs vitamin E and canthaxantin. In Eggs and Eggs Products Quality, Proceedings of VIII European Symposium on the Quality of Eggs and Egg Products, vol II. Bologna, Italy, Sept. 19–23, 1999.
49. Elwinger, K., and Inborr, J. 1999. Composition and taste of eggs enriched with omega-3 fatty acids and natural astaxanthin. In Eggs and Eggs Products Quality, Proceedings of VIII European Symposium on the Quality of Eggs and Egg Products, vol. II. Bologna, Italy, 1999, Sept. 19–23, 1999.
50. Mozzon, M., Ruggieri, S., and Frega, N. 1999. Study on the fatty acid composition of eggs produced by hens fed with n-3 fatty acid-enriched feed. In Eggs and Eggs Products Quality, Proceedings of VIII European Symposium on the Quality of Eggs and Egg Products, vol. II. Bologna, Italy, Sept. 19–23, 1999.
51. Farrel, D.J. 1992. The fortification of hens' eggs with omega-3 long chain fatty acids and their effect in humans. International Symposium on Nonconventional Eggs Uses and Newly Emerging Processing Technologies. Banff Springs Hotel, Banff, Alberta, Canada, Apr. 1992.
52. Zhin Bin, Huang, Loibovitz, H., Lee, C.M., and Millar, R. 1990. Effect of dietary fish oil, on n-3 fatty acid levels in chicken eggs and thigh flesh. J Agric Food Chem 38:743–47.
53. Herber, S.M. Dietary marine algae promotes efficient deposition of n-3 fatty acids for the production of enriched shell eggs. Poult Sci 1996;75(12):1501–7.
54. Herber, S.M., and Van Elswyk, M.E. Dietary marine algae maintains egg consumer acceptability while enhancing yolk color. Poult Sci 1998;77(3):493–96.
55. Carrillo, S., Carranco, M.E., Castillo, R.M., Castro-González, M.I., Pérez-Gil, F., and Avila, E. El huevo como fuente de acidos grasos n-3 y n-6 al incorporar harina del crustáceo langostilla en raciones para ponedoras. XVI Congreso Latinoamericano de Avicultura, septiembre. Lima, Perú, 1999, pp. 338–42.
56. Beyer, R.S., and Jensen, L.S. Influence of orotic acid on performance, liver lipid content and egg cholesterol level of laying hens. Poult Sci 1991;70(11):2322–28.
57. Leeson, S., Caston, L.J., and Summers, J.D. Response of laying hens to supplemental niacin. Poult Sci 1991;70(5):1231–35.
58. Beyer, R.S., and Jensen, L.S. Cholesterol concentration of egg yolk and blood plasma and performance of laying hens as influenced by dietary alpha ketoisocaproic acid. Poult Sci 1992;71(1):170–72.
59. Hargis, P.S. Modifying egg yolk cholesterol in the domestic fowl: a review. World's Poult Sci J 1988;44:17–29.
60. Albala, C., García, C., Yañez, M., and Jury, G. Influencia del consumo de huevos sobre el perfil lipídico en hombres adultos sanos. Rev Chil Nutr 1996;24(2):103–13.

61. Schnorr, P., Thomsen, O.O., Riis-Hansen, P., Boberg-Ans, G., Lawaetz, H., and Weeke, T. Egg consumption and high density lipoprotein cholesterol. J Intern Med 1994;235:249–51.
62. Oh, S.Y., Ryue, J., Hsieh, C.H., and Bell, D.E. Eggs enriched in omega-3 fatty acids and alterations in lipid concentrations in plasma and lipoproteins and blood pressure. Am J Clin Nutr 1991;54:689–95.
63. United States Department of Agriculture. USDA. Dietary Guidelines for Americans 2000. 5th Edition, 2000. http://www.nal.usda.gov/fnic/dga.

16

Predictability of Respiratory Atopy from Egg Hypersensitivity in Children

Kelly Blackstock

Basic Mechanisms of an Allergic Reaction

The body's ability to combat disease comes from the immune functions of the lymphatic system. Resistance to pathogens is divided into specific and nonspecific. Nonspecific resistance is made up of general mechanisms of attack directed toward a variety of foreign invaders. Specific resistance involves specialized lymphocytes recognizing a particular pathogen. This branch of immunity mediates allergic responses. Typical lymphocytes associated with specific resistance are B-cells and T-cells, although mast cells and basophils are synergists in subsequent reactivity.

Substances that elicit reactivity are called antigens. Antigens become introduced into the body through the respiratory tract or gastrointestinal tract or through contact of the integument. Initial contact of an antigen to a predisposed person will not manifest symptoms; rather, the immune system will become *sensitized*. Sensitization begins with recognition of a specific antigen by a matching B cell. Antigen protein will be presented on the plasma membrane of the B-cell by the major histocompatibility complex (MHC). Corresponding T-cells, once bound to the MHC, will release chemicals, stimulating the B-cell to divide. The final result of B-cell division is the production of antibodies, or immunoglobins (Igs). The binding sites of the Igs will be specific for the initial antigen. Several isotopes of Igs exist, but it is IgE that is responsible for allergic hypersensitivity. Once the immune system has become sensitized, it is primed to react to a second exposure. Circulating IgEs will bind to new antigens and then to the F_c receptors of both mast cells and basophils. Following binding, mast cells and basophils are stimulated to produce histamine and prostaglandin, whose actions include promoting inflammation and other clinical allergic symptoms.

All true allergies are manifested through this mechanism. However, it should be noted that a variety of IgEs exist for the array of possible antigens. For this reason differences arise between allergies in their expression. Factors including age, gender, ethnicity, stress, and seasonal changes can affect when and if an individual will be sensitive to an antigen.[2,15] For example, aeroallergens typically affect individuals later in life, while food allergens prevail in infancy.[9,15]

Food Allergy

Food allergies are generically described as adverse reactions to food generated by an immune response. Food antigens are water-soluble, heat- and acid-stable glycoproteins with molecular weights between 15 and 60 kDa.[1] Their admittance to the body is through the GI tract (although studies have shown reactivity to food as aeroallergens).[9] For any immunologic reaction to occur, there must first be penetration of molecules through a barrier, in this case the mucosal membrane of the intestines. It has been demonstrated in studies as early as the 1930s that antigenically intact macromolecules are transmitted across the mammalian gut. Wilson and Walzer intradurally injected IgE antibodies specific for hen eggs in both adult and juvenile subjects. Upon ingestion of eggs, an average of 79.7 percent of subjects had positive reactions, proving significant intestinal absorption.[16]

Though antigen absorption does exist, it should be minimal, making reactivity almost nonexistent. It is the role of the mucosa, specifically a protein called secretory immunoglobin A (sIgA), to act as a barrier and prevent a majority of macromolecule absorption from occurring. Transient deficiencies in sIgA have been linked to reagenic manifestations.[14] Injury, inheritance, or immaturity typically causes defects in the barrier.[2] In the case of children, immaturity appears to be the most prominent contributor to food allergy. It is hypothesized that immature sIgA in children allows more antigenic protein to cross over, compounding any predisposition.[2,15] This assumption is validated by the fact that food allergy is the most common allergen in the first years of life[10,11,15] and decreases in occurrence with age.

Egg Hypersensitivity

Of all food allergens, egg appears to be the most common.[1,9,10,12,15,17,18] Egg protein, or albumen, was found to be more allergenic than the yolk.[15] Albumen constituents include ovalbumin (54 percent), ovatransferrin (12 percent), and ovomucoid (11 percent). Ovomucoid is most often associated with allergic responses because of its thermostability and resistance to trypsin digestion. Severity of reaction is dependent on the individual. Minute exposure to egg protein can be mild or result in life-threatening anaphylaxis.[1]

Treatment of egg allergy, as with all food allergies, is a restrictive diet. Concerns do arise involving nutrient deficiencies, especially with children, but eggs are not a primary source of any one nutrient. Their exclusion, then, poses no nutritional threat.[4] Egg-sensitive individuals usually have greater difficulties isolating the hidden sources of eggs. Binders, emulsifiers, coagulants, and clarifying agents are just a few roles that egg components play in food preparation. For this reason eggs can be found in items as innocuous as root beer, salad dressing, soups, candy, and meat products.[1,4,15] In addition, cross contamination of foods during restaurant preparation is common. Cooking rarely helps because egg allergens are recognized by human serum IgE even after pasteurization.[8] Furthermore, many vaccines, including influenza, yellow fever, and typhus, are harvested in chick embryo tissues, posing yet another concern.

Connection of Food Allergy to Respiratory Atopy

Prevalence of atopic disorders, including atopic dermatitis, urticaria, and asthma, has been steadily rising in children.[5] For this reason, increasing interest has been directed toward isolating predictive measures so that primary and secondary interventions can be initiated. Though controversial, some researchers believe early sensitization to any antigen results in an increased risk of developing subsequent allergic disease.[5,6,13,17] Prediction, then, would be most valuable during gestation or in early infancy. Attempts at finding a prenatal marker using umbilical cord levels of total IgE, however, proved unfounded.[6,10,12,17] New theories have surfaced using indicator markers that develop promptly postnatally, the most common being total serum IgE and specific IgE to food antigens.

The majority of investigation into total serum IgE has been done by Kulig et al. In a recent study involving 4,082 German children, these researchers evaluated serum IgE levels in atopic versus nonatopic children annually from birth until 6 years of age. As was hypothesized, IgE percentiles were markedly higher in atopic versus nonatopic subjects ($p < 0.001$). Distributions were graphed and found to overlap considerably, making a discernable division between atopic and nonatopic children impossible. The inability to discriminate between atopic and nonatopic children reflects the moderate capacity of total IgE as a reliable predictor.[7] Similar findings were reported by Zeiger and Heller and again by Kulig et al.[18,5]

Another shift in investigation is toward the use of food allergens as predictors. IgE antibodies against inhalant allergies usually appear later in life among allergic individuals in comparison with IgE antibodies against food allergens, which appear in infancy. The apparent inverse proportionality between time of development of respiratory and food allergens might suggest a physiological link. Early theories connecting the two are predominantly circumstantial. The first hypothesized connection is that ingested allergens are found to circulate quickly to nasal mucosa, stimulating mast cells to increase airway reactivity. Also, asthma can be exacerbated by inhalation of airborne food proteins.[15] The relation of reactivity could possibly indicate that IgE antibodies are not entirely specific to only one antigen, suggesting that cross-reactivity is occurring. Secondly, food-sensitized children are more prone to aeroallergens,[2,5,6,10] and aeroallergens are linked to atopy such as asthma.[5,12] At least one study has confirmed the connection, showing children with food allergies at age 7 years to have almost two times the prevalence of both allergic rhinitis and asthma compared with those without food allergies.[18]

Of all food allergens studied, specific IgE to egg protein had the highest correlation to atopic disease.[6,5,10,12,18] Sigurs et al. showed that of 135 subjects with at least one food allergen, 46 had significant levels (0.35 kU/L) of IgE to eggs. Of those egg-sensitive individuals, 57 percent had developed aeroallergens by 2 years of age and 76 percent by 15 years of age.[13] Additional studies found that not only was egg sensitivity significantly linked to atopy including asthma but also risk of development of atopic disease in those high-risk infants was at least doubled by age 7.[2,17]

Evidence regarding degree of sensitization has compounded the issue. Findings showed early sensitization leading to higher concentrations of serum IgE to egg protein.[6,10] Consequently, varying levels of concentration were evaluated as risk predictors. It appears that as serum levels of IgE increase so does risk. Going one step further, studies showed children with long-lasting sensitization developed allergic rhinitis and allergic asthma significantly more often than children just transiently sensitized to egg protein. ($p < .001$), increasing the risk of allergic rhinitis 3.4 times and asthma 5.5 times.[6] However, these findings are controversial. Prophylactic procedures done by Zeiger and Heller showed no relationship of food sensitization to development of atopy.[18]

Is Egg IgE a Valuable Predictor?

Correlation tied to egg IgE was high in all studies, but to be an accurate predictor, clinical sensitivity and positive predictive values (PPVs) also need to be high. In most cases use of specific IgE to eggs increased both the sensitivity and PPV;[5,6,10,12] however, the highest recorded sensitivity was 56 percent (Table 16.1). This means that, of all individuals that will develop atopy, the IgE egg marker will only detect 56 percent of them. The highest PPV (71 percent) still leaves a 29 percent chance of false-positives. The strength of the IgE egg marker lies in the clinical specificity, ranging from 92 to 97 percent. Unfortunately, this information is of little use to prevention.

Lack of validity for egg IgE as a predictor led some researchers to cross-examine the marker with other variables. Family history and risk profiles were evaluated most often.[5,9,12,18] By themselves, they too were poor predictors of atopy, but together with egg IgE, they drastically increased sensitivity and PPV. One study showed PPV rising from 37 to 70 percent, and another listed sensitivity as high as 86 percent with the inclusion of a positive family history.[5,10]

The appeal of using food-specific antibody to determine risks of atopic development is understandable. The tests are easy to perform and cost-effective. The greater challenge is obtaining high enough results for clinical sensitivity and PPV. As of yet, egg-specific IgE tests are not sufficient for predicting atopic disorders. Furthermore, critics contend that previously obtained results were biased, arising from homogeneous cohorts of genetically high-risk subjects. Inclusion of additional members of a more general population could warrant a decrease in predictability percentages, although of the articles that were reviewed most implemented large cohorts. Also, allergenicity was determined and compared by both skin-prick tests and radioallergosorbent test (RAST), neither of which is without limitations. Sensitization, however, is a prerequisite for development of allergic airway disease.[6,5,9] Sensitized children must be regarded as high risk for subsequent development of allergic disease, a fact noted by strong correlation and relatively high sensitivity. For these reasons, the IgE egg marker for respiratory atopy should not be abandoned. Rather, further study should be implemented not only for specific egg IgE as a predictor but also to unravel the physiological mechanism that might link the two.

Table 16.1. Capacity of egg sensitization to predict the development of respiratory atopy

Study	Risk factor	Sensitivity (%)	Specificity (%)	PPV (%)
Hattevig et al.[a,*]	8-mo egg-IgE ≥ 0.35 kU/L	56	96	63
Nickel et al.[b,*]	1-yr egg-IgE ≥ 0.35 kU/L	20	93	36
Zeiger and Heller[c,*]	Egg-IgE skin-prick test (1-yr)	21	93	80
Kulig et al.[d,*]	1-yr egg-IgE ≥ 0.35 kU/L	35	94	71

Note. PPV = positive predictive value.
[a]Reference 3.
[b]Reference 10.
[c]Reference 18.
[d]Reference 6.
[*]$P < .001$

REFERENCES

1. Breneman, J.C. Handbook of Food Allergies. New York: M. Decker, 1987.
2. Burr, M.L., Merrett, T.G., Dunstan, F.D., and Maguire, M.J. The development of allergy in high-risk children. Clin Exp Allergy 1997;27(11):1247–53.
3. Hattevig, G., Kjellman, B., and Bjorksten, B. Clinical symptoms and IgE responses to common food proteins and inhalants in the first 7 years of life. Clin Allergy, Nov. 1987;17(6):571–78.
4. Koerner, C.B., and Hays, T.L. Food Allergy: Current Knowledge and Future Directions. Immunology and Allergy Clinics of North America, Aug. 1999;19(3):583–603.
5. Kulig, M., Bergman, R., Niggemann, B., Burow, G., Wahn, U., and the MAS Study Group. Prediction of sensitization to inhalant allergens in childhood: evaluating family history, atopic dermatitis and food sensitization to food allergens. Clin Exp Allergy, Nov. 1998:28(11):1397–1403.
6. Kulig, M., Bergman, R., Tacke, U., Wahn, U., and Guggenmoos-Holzman, I. Long-lasting sensitization to food during the first two years precedes allergic airway disease. Pediatr Allergy Immunol 1998;9:61–67.
7. Kulig, M., Tacke, U., Forster, J., Edenharter, G., Bergmann, R., Lau, S., Wahn, V., Zepp, F., Wahn, U., and the MAS Study Group. Serum IgE levels during the first 6 years of life. J Pediatr, Apr. 1999;134(4):453–58.
8. Leduc, V., Demeulemester, C., Polack, B., Guizard, C., Le Guern, L., and Peltre, G.. Immunochemical detection of egg-white antigens and allergens in meat products. Allergy 1999;54:464–72.

9. Metcalfe, D., Sampson, H.A., and Simon R.A. Food Allergy: Adverse Reactions to Foods and Food Additives. Cambridge, MA: Blackwell Science, 1997.
10. Nickel, R., Kulig, M., Forster, J., Bergman, R., Bauer, C.P., Lau, S., Guggenmoos-Holzman, I., and Wahn U. Sensitization to hen's egg at the age of twelve months is predictive for allergic sensitization to common indoor and outdoor allergens at the age of three years. J Allergy Clin Immunol, May 1997;99(5):613–17.
11. Sampson, H.A. Relationship between food-specific IgE concentrations and the risk of positive food challenges in children and adolescents. J Allergy Clin Immunol 1997;100:444–51.
12. Sasai, K., Furukawa, S., Muto, T., Baba, M., Yabuta, K., and Fukuwatari, Y. Early detection of specific IgE antibody against house dust mite in children at risk of allergic disease. J Pediatr, June 1996;128(6):834–40.
13. Sigurs, N., Hattevig, G., Kjellman, B., Kjellman, N.I., Nilsson, L., and Bjorksten, B. Appearance of atopic disease in relation to serum IgE antibodies in children followed up from birth for 4 to 15 years. J Allergy Clin Immunol, Oct. 1994;94(4):757–63.
14. Soothill, J.F., Stokes, R., Turner, M.W., Norman, A.P., and Taylor, B. Predisposing factors and the development of reaginic allergy in infancy. Clin Allergy 1976;6:305–19.
15. Trevino, R.J. Food Allergy. New York: Thieme, 1997.
16. Wilson, S., and Walzer, M. Absorption of undigested proteins in human beings: IV. Absorption of unaltered egg protein in infants and in children. Am J Dis Child 1929;10:40–54.
17. Yunginger, J.W., Ahlstedt, S., Eggleston, P.A., Homburger, H.A., Nelson, H.S., Ownby, D.R., Platts-Mills, T., Sampson, H.A., Sichcer, S.H., Weinstein, A.M., Williams, P.B., Wood, R.A., and Zeiger, R.S. Quantitative IgE antibody assays in allergic diseases. J Allergy Clin Immunol, June 2000;105(6):1077–84.
18. Zeiger, R.S., and Heller, S. The development and prediction of atopy in high-risk children: follow-up at age seven years in a prospective randomized study of combined maternal and infant food allergen avoidance. J Allergy Clin Immunol, June 1995;95(6):1179–90.

17

Effects of Cooking and Storage on the Nutritional Value of Eggs

Giorgio Bedogni
and Nino Carlo Battistini

Introduction

"And to this research and discovery which name more appropriate than Medicine could be given? Because this discovery was made for the health of man, for his salvation and feeding, in place of that regimen from which troubles, diseases and death were coming":[1] this is how the author of *De Antica Medicina*—the most famous treatise of the *Corpus Hippocraticum*—heralds the discovery of cooking, which, in his account, marked the beginning of medicine. Even if nowadays such an assertion is considered exaggerated, there is some truth in it. Apart from making foods more digestible, cooking actually increases the availability of some minerals (e.g., iron).[2] However, cooking may also reduce the content of some nutrients, especially vitamins.[3,4] Storage is another "discovery" of humans that has substantially improved their food intake. However, storage may also produce loss of nutrients.[3] This chapter offers a brief critical review of the effects of cooking and storage on the nutritional value of the hen egg.

Eggs in Nutrition

We start by recalling the main nutritional properties of eggs since this will allow us to better understand the effects of cooking and storage on their nutritional value. First, eggs are sources of high-quality proteins (and are in fact the standard against which the protein quality of other foods is judged). Second, eggs are rich in unsaturated fatty acids. Third, eggs are rich in cholesterol and are sources of many vitamins and minerals (Table 17.1).

Effects of Cooking on the Nutrient Content of Eggs

To explain the effects of cooking, we compared the nutrient content of raw eggs with that of boiled, fried, poached, and scrambled eggs using the data provided by the Royal Chemistry Society.[6] The egg samples and the recipes employed to produce these data are described in Table 17.2.

Table 17.1. Contribution of a 100 g hen egg to the recommended daily allowance (RDA) of vitamins and minerals for an adult man (25–50 years)

	Qty. / 100 g	RDA (%)
Vitamin B_{12} (μg)	2.50	125
Biotin (μg)	20.00	20–67[a]
Panthotenic acid (mg)	1.77	25–44[a]
Iodine (μg)	53.00	35
Vitamin D (μg)	1.75	35
Riboflavin (mg)	0.47	28
Folic acid (μg)	50.00	25
Retinol (μg)	190.00	19
Iron (mg)	1.90	19
Phosphorus (mg)	200.00	17
Vitamin E (mg)	1.11	11

Source. Values were calculated from the egg composition provided by the Royal Chemistry Society[6] and the RDA for Americans.[5]

Note. Only micronutrients with a contribution > 10 percent are given.

[a]Variability within the recommended range.

Table 17.2. Egg samples and recipes employed to develop the egg composition tables of the Royal Chemistry Society

Raw (whole) egg	Analysis of battery, deep litter and free range
Boiled egg	10 eggs
Fried egg (vegetable oil)	12 eggs, shallow fried
Poached egg	10 eggs, no fat added
Scrambled egg (milk)	2 eggs, 20 g butter, 15 ml milk, ½ level tsp. salt; melt butter in pan, stir in beaten egg, milk, and seasoning. Cook over gentle heat until moisture thickens.

Source. Reference 6.

Note. Allowances were made for any water loss or fat uptake in cases where eggs were cooked with fat.

Macronutrients

Boiling and poaching have virtually no effect on eggs' macronutrient content (Table 17.3). However, both frying and scrambling substantially increase their energy value through the addition of fats. Scrambling may be responsible for a modest loss of proteins. However, the intestinal absorption of egg proteins and their accumulation in body tissues is greater for cooked than for raw eggs. For instance, Evenepoel et al. recently showed that 94 percent (25 g) of cooked egg proteins are assimilated as compared with 64 percent of (the same amount of) raw proteins.[7]

Boiling and poaching were found not to be associated with any change in lipid composition (Table 17.4), which was confirmed by previous observations.[8] Of course, the addition of oil for frying does increase fatty acids and that of butter is responsible for a substantial increase in saturated fatty acids in scrambled eggs.

Micronutrients

Vitamins

Owing to their susceptibility to thermal degradation,[9] water-soluble vitamins are the micronutrients of egg most prone to loss during cooking (Table 17.5).

According to data provided by the Royal Chemistry Society, vitamin B_{12} undergoes the greatest average loss (42 percent) (Fig. 17.1), with a substantial difference, however, between scrambling (16 percent) and boiling (56 percent). Riboflavin, pantothenic acid, folic acid, thiamin, and biotin are lost in amounts between 18 and 28 percent, while pyridoxine and niacin are virtually unmodified. As noted by Everson and Souders[10] and reviewed by Froning,[11] the loss of thiamin is independent of the cooking method employed. However, contrary to what Hanning reported,[11,12] similar losses of riboflavin take place in scrambling and boiling. Moreover, according to these data, the susceptibility of folic acid to undergo loss appears to be lower than reputed in the past.[11] As far as folic acid is concerned, it should be noted that egg (yolk) folates are the most stable and bioavailable among many foods.[13]

Finally, the data of the Royal Chemistry Society show that among liposoluble vitamins (A, E, and D) only vitamin D undergoes a modest loss in scrambled eggs.

Table 17.3. Effect of cooking on the macronutrient and energy content of eggs

	Raw	Boiled (% change)	Fried (% change)	Poached (% change)	Scrambled (% change)
Proteins (g%)	12.5	0	+ 9	0	−14
Fats (g%)	10.8	0	+29	0	+109
Carbohydrates (g%)	Tr	Tr	Tr	Tr	Tr
Energy (kJ)	612.0	0	+22	0	+67

Source. Percent changes were calculated from the data of the Royal Chemistry Society.
Note. Tr = tracks.

Table 17.4. Effect of cooking on the fatty acid profile of eggs

	Raw	Boiled (% change)	Fried (% change)	Poached (% change)	Scrambled (% change)
SFA (g / 100 g)	3.1	0	+ 29	0	+274
MUFA (g / 100 g)	4.7	0	+ 28	0	+ 53
PUFA (g / 100 g)	1.2	0	+ 25	0	+ 17

Source. Percent changes were calculated from the data of the Royal Chemistry Society.[6]
Note. SFA = saturated fatty acid; MUFA = monounsaturated fatty acid; PUFA = polyunsaturated fatty acid.

Table 17.5. Effect of cooking on the vitamin content of eggs

	Raw	Boiled (% change)	Fried (% change)	Poached (% change)	Scrambled (% change)
Thiamin (mg / 100 g)	0.09	−22	−22	−22	−22
Riboflavin (mg / 100 g)	0.47	−25	−34	−23	−30
Niacin (mg / 100 g)	0.10	0	0	0	0
Pyridoxine (mg / 100 g)	0.12	0	+17	0	−25
Biotin (μg / 100 g)	20.00	−20	−10	−25	−17
Pantothenic acid (mg / 100 g)	1.77	−26	−26	−26	−27
Folic acid (mg / 100 g)	50.00	−22	−20[a]	−10	−44
Vitamin B_{12} (μg / 100 g)	2.50	−56	−36	−60	−16
Vitamin C (mg / 100 g)	0	0	0	0	Tr
Vitamin A (μg / 100 g)	190.00	Tr	+13	0	+55
Carotene (μg / 100 g)[b]	Tr	Tr	Tr	Tr	Tr
Vitamin D (μg / 100 g)[c]	1.75	0	+14	0[a]	−11
Vitamin E (μg / 100 g)	1.11	0	N/A	0	+11

Source. Percent changes were calculated from the data of the Royal Chemistry Society.[6]
Note. Tr = tracks; N/A = not available.
[a]Estimated value.
[b]Given as β-carotene equivalents.
[c]Values may be higher for hens fed a supplement.

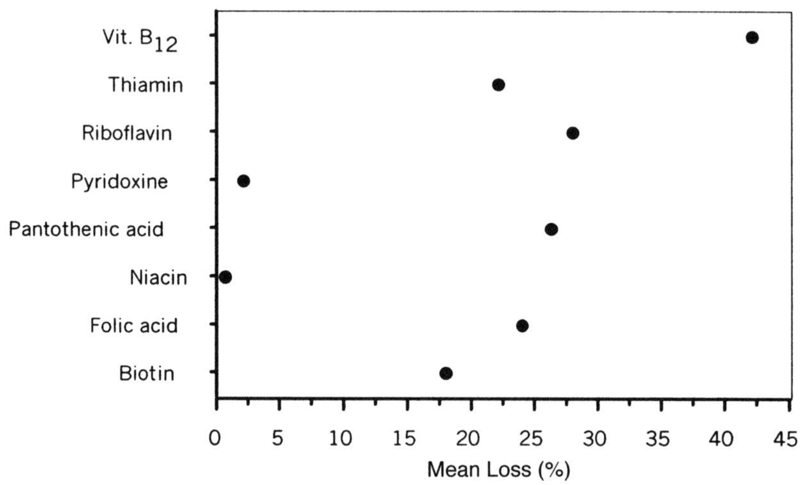

Figure 17.1. Mean losses of egg water-soluble vitamins during cooking. The graph was drawn from the data presented in Table 17.5.

Minerals

Boiling and poaching do not affect the mineral content of eggs (Table 17.6). Many minerals undergo a modest increase in percentage as a result of frying, and the addition of salt for scrambled eggs does substantially increase the quantity of sodium and chloride. Modest losses of phosphorus, iron, copper, zinc, selenium, and iodine occur with scrambling. However, it should be noted that iron's bioavailability actually increases with cooking.[14]

Table 17.6. Effect of cooking on the mineral content of eggs

	Raw	Boiled (% change)	Fried (% change)	Poached (% change)	Scrambled (% change)
Sodium (mg / 100 g)	140	0	+14	0	+636
Potassium (mg / 100 g)	130	0	+15	0	0
Calcium (mg / 100 g)	57	0	+14	0	+11
Magnesium (mg / 100 g)	12	0	+17	0	+42
Phosphorus (mg / 100 g)	200	0	+15	0	−10
Iron (mg / 100 g)	1.9	0	+16	0	−16
Copper (mg / 100 g)	0.08	0	+12	0	−12
Zinc (mg / 100 g)	1.3	0	+15	0	−15
Chloride (mg / 100 g)	160	0	+12	0	+869
Manganese (mg / 100 g)	Tr	Tr	Tr	Tr	Tr
Selenium (μg / 100 g)	11	0	+ 9	0	−18
Iodine (μg / 100 g)	53	0	+13	0	− 2

Source. Percent changes were calculated from the data of the Royal Chemistry Society.[6]
Note. Tr = tracks.

EFFECTS OF STORAGE ON THE NUTRIENT CONTENT OF EGGS

Cold storage is reported not to produce substantial modifications of the protein content of eggs.[11] As far as lipids are concerned, no consistent changes in fatty acid content of shell eggs were seen after cold storage at 0°C for 6 to 12 months.[8] Studies of cold storage of eggs have shown significant losses of pyridoxine already at 3 months; increasing losses of riboflavin, niacin, pyridoxine, and folic acid at 6 months; and more significant losses of pyridoxine, folic acid, and vitamin B_{12} at 12 months (Table 17.7).[11] Apparently, pantothenic acid and biotin are minimally affected by cold storage. For most vitamins, however, losses are relevant only after 3 months of storage, and since eggs are presently marketed within a few days, these losses are probably of no practical relevance.

Table 17.7. Effect of cold storage on the vitamin content of eggs

	Raw	3 months (% change)	6 months (% change)	12 months (% change)
Riboflavin (μg / g)	3.49	5	16	12
Niacin (mg / g)	0.66	9	18	N/A
Pyridoxine (μg / g)	2.52	18	29	47
Biotin (ng / g)	225.00	0 (−8)[a]	0 (2)[a]	0 (−1)[a]
Pantothenic acid (μg / g)	12.50	6	6	6
Folic acid (ng / g)	94.00	1	15	21
Vit. B_{12} (ng / g)	6.54	7	6	23

Source. Data were adapted from Froning[11] with minor modifications (percent values were recalculated from raw data).
Note. N/A = not available.
[a]The values between parentheses were considered equivalent to zero.

Dehydrated eggs do not generally show protein losses, and their content of riboflavin and niacin is stable.[11] However, significant losses in retinol have been described. These losses are due to oxidation and are more significant at high storage temperatures. For example, 9 months of storage at –9.4°C resulted in a 60 percent loss; at 21.1°C, a 75 percent loss; and at 37.0°C, an 80 percent loss.[11] Dehydration does not appear to influence substantially the baseline vitamin D content of eggs.[11]

Conclusion

Based on this review, the following conclusions can be drawn about the effects of cooking and storage on the nutritional values of eggs:

- Among cooking methods for eggs, scrambling may be responsible for a loss of proteins. However, this loss is modest and does not change the fact that the hen is a rich source of proteins.
- Boiling and poaching are preferable to scrambling because they do not add fats, which increase the energy value of eggs and alter the fatty acid profile of the hen egg. This is not to say that the consumption of scrambled eggs should be avoided by healthy individuals but, simply, that scrambling should be less frequently employed than other forms of cooking to better safeguard the nutritional value of eggs as far as their lipid composition is concerned.
- The fact that vitamin B_{12} may be lost at values as high as 60 percent (poaching) when eggs are cooked does not change the fact that eggs are a rich source of this vitamin. In fact, even with a loss of 60 percent, a 100 g poached egg would still be able to contribute 50 percent of the adult Recommended Daily Allowance for vitamin B_{12}. Losses of other water-soluble vitamins are lower and are expected to be counteracted by eating a balanced diet rich in fruits and vegetables. Among liposoluble vitamins only vitamin D undergoes a modest loss.
- Losses in minerals due to cooking are generally low and are expected to be counteracted by eating a balanced diet rich in fruits and vegetables.
- Cold storage affects the vitamin content of eggs only after long periods (≥3 months), a circumstance that is quite uncommon with actual marketing channels.

Thus, the nutritional value of the cooked egg, especially when boiled or fried with vegetable oil, is high and confirms that hen eggs are a nutritious and healthy food.

References

1. De Antica Medicina, c. 3 (translation by authors). Littré, Ouvres complètes, 10 vols. Paris 1839–1861.
2. Lee, K., and Clydesdale, F.M. Effect of thermal processing on endogenous and added iron in canned spinach. J Food Sci 1981;46:1064.
3. Severi, S., Bedogni, G., Manzieri, A.M., et al. Effects of cooking and storage methods on the micronutrient content of foods. Eur J Cancer Prev 1997;6(Suppl. 1):S21.

4. Severi, S., Bedogni, G., Zoboli, G.P., et al. Effects of home-based food preparation practices on the micronutrient content of foods. Eur J Cancer Prev 1998;7:331.
5. Food and Nutrition Board. Recommended Dietary Allowances. Washington, DC: National Academy Press, 1989.
6. Holland, B., Welch, A.A., Unwin, I.D., et al. McCance and Widdowson's the Composition of Foods. Cambridge: Royal Society of Chemistry, 1994.
7. Evenepoel, P., Claus, D., Geypens, B., et al. Amount and fate of egg protein escaping assimilation in the small intestine of humans. Am J Physiol 1999;277:G935.
8. Posati, L.P., Kinsella, J.E., Watt, B.K. Comprehensive evaluation of fatty acids in foods. III. Eggs and egg products, J Am Dietet Assoc 1975;67:111.
9. Harris, R.S. General discussion on the stability of nutrients. In Nutritional Evaluation of Food Processing, Karmas, E., and Harris, R.S., eds. New York: Van Nostrand Reinold Company, 1988, chap. 1.
10. Everson, G.J., and Souders, H.J. Composition and nutritive importance of eggs. J Am Diet Assoc 1957;33:1244.
11. Froning, G.W. Effects of agricultural practices on poultry and eggs. In Nutrition and Evaluation of Food Processing, Karmas, E., and Harris, R.S., eds. New York: Van Nostrand Reinold Company, 1988, chap. 9.
12. Hanning, F. The effect of a plastic coating of shell eggs on changes which occur during storage and cooking. Poult Sci 1957;36:1365.
13. Seyoum, E., and Selhub, J. Properties of food folates determined by stability and susceptibility to intestinal pteroylpolyglutamate hydrolase action. J Nutr 1998;128:1956.
14. Miller, J., and Nnanna, I. Bioavailability of iron in cooked egg yolk for maintenance of hemoglobin levels in growing rats. J Nutr 1983;113:1169.

18

The Potential Use of Eggs for the Protein Requirements of Endurance Exercise

Jaclyn Maurer

Introduction

Athletic excellence is a must for any serious athlete. Attaining this excellence is a complicated process that includes proper training, adequate rest, and a balanced diet. Numerous studies have been conducted exploring the carbohydrate requirements of and optimal carbohydrate sources for endurance athletes, leaving other nutrients like protein in the background. Existing and emerging research, however, is introducing the possibility of increasing protein requirements for endurance athletes based on the body's changing needs for protein during endurance exercise. The best sources of protein to satisfy these needs are still unclear; however, egg protein lends itself as a potentially optimal choice of protein for endurance athletes.

Our Basic Need for Protein

Before one can understand why exercise may increase the body's need for dietary protein, it is critical to understand why the body needs dietary protein to begin with. Essentially, protein is responsible for regulation of gene expression; biochemical catalysts; formation of major cellular structural elements: muscle, nails, teeth, hair, ligaments; and formation of antibodies and hormones.[1] The building blocks of protein are amino acids. Twenty amino acids exist; some are nonessential (our body can synthesize them), while nine are essential and can only be obtained from dietary protein intake.[2] When ingested in the diet, synthesized via excess carbohydrates or fat and ammonia, or released from the breakdown of our own body proteins, these amino acids will enter the body's pools of free amino acids.[3] The amino acids in these pools are then utilized for protein synthesis and called upon to compensate for the breakdown of body protein. The breakdown of body protein happens readily with exercise and is discussed in the following sections.

Adequate dietary protein intake is necessary to keep the pools full of free amino acids (both essential and nonessential) for the body to utilize as needed. When dietary protein intake is compromised or poor, the body starts to deplete the free amino acids in its pools. As the pools empty and do not get replenished, losses in muscle size and strength can occur, since amino acids are being drawn from the muscles to refill these pools.[3] These decreases will eventually lead to fatigue and weaker performance in physically active people. Clearly, adequate protein intake is necessary for our bodies to perform at their optimum physically.

Physical Activity and Our Need for Protein

Muscle activity over a prolonged time (i.e., endurance exercise) causes exercise-induced muscle injury (structural damage to muscle) and increases in mitochondrial protein synthesis. This structural damage to muscle invokes protein synthesis as a means of repair, while an increase in mitochondrial protein synthesis promotes amino acid oxidation.[2,4,5] As the body demands more ATP production to fuel working muscles during endurance exercise, the muscles start to utilize amino acids for this needed fuel.[2]

Initially, the liver regulates amino acids from ingested protein; however, the liver does not control the fate of branch chain amino acids (BCAAs). Instead BCAAs travel to the adipose and muscle tissue and are metabolized as needed. The presence of enzymes specific to the catabolism of BCAA—like the enzyme branch chain α-keto acid dehydrogenase (BCKA dehydrogenase), which controls the irreversible decarboxylation of BCAAs, primarily in the muscle—supports the hypothesis that amino acids may be used as a direct fuel source for muscle.[1,2] Both amino acid oxidation and exercise-induced muscle injury increase protein metabolism. This ties back to the body's need for ample pools of free amino acids to pull from in order to offset the protein degradation and amino acid oxidation that endurance exercise induces. It is important to note, however, that the extent of amino acid oxidation and muscle structural damage is suggested to be dependent on the intensity and duration of the exercise.[2–5] According to findings from Lemon, the limiting enzyme BCKA dehydrogenase is dependent on the intensity and duration of exercise.[4] Researchers Kasperek and Snider supported Lemon's finding with their research that discovered the activity of BCKA dehydrogenase increased as the intensity of exercise increased.[6] Kasperek and Snider linked this increase to an increased requirement for citric acid cycle intermediates.[6] (Note that intermediates for the citric acid cycle are readily utilized during endurance exercise as the need for the generation of ATP increases.) Additional research has documented that mild-intensity endurance exercise will increase amino acid oxidation, but this increase is balanced throughout the day via times of reduced oxidation.[2] Thus, while endurance exercise does appear to increase protein requirements, the extent of this increased need is related to the intensity of the exercise.[4] Therefore, going for a leisurely jog will promote amino acid oxidation but less than a prolonged, intense tempo run. This is an important point for an endurance athlete to consider since it requires the athlete to monitor and adjust protein intake according to training duration and intensity.

Interestingly, research of amino acid oxidation and endurance exercise led to the discovery that the synthesis of the amino acid alanine in the muscle greatly increased with increased exercise intensity. It was found that as both exercise intensity and amino acid oxidation increased, the synthesis of alanine in the muscle greatly increased to help minimize the accumulation of muscle pyruvate. (Alanine is synthesized via the transfer of the amino group from BCAAs to the carbon of pyruvate, and thus the amount of pyruvate produced in the muscle is decreased.[5] Alanine also serves as a means for transporting the nitrogen from the catabolism of amino acids to the liver for disposal. Once in the liver, this alanine can be converted to glucose and released into the bloodstream where it is picked up and utilized by muscle for energy.[1]) By minimizing the production of muscle pyruvate, the synthesis of alanine in intense working muscles helps offset the production of lactate and consequently wards off fatigue.[5] This finding suggests that branch chain amino acids could potentially be useful as fuel for endurance exercise.

Furthermore, a study done by Hayward et al. examining the effects in rats of dietary protein on enzyme activity after exercise showed that the amount of dietary protein consumed greatly affected both muscle and serum enzyme activity.[7] The enzymes creatine kinase, lactate dehydrogenase, pyruvate kinase, and aspartate aminotransferase come from the skeletal muscle. An increase of these enzymes in the serum following exercise indicates muscle injury. Ideally, an athlete would want to reduce the release of these enzymes after exercise to reduce muscle injury, and Hayward et al. hypothesized that an increase in dietary protein would do that. However, all they found was that rats fed high-protein diets and engaging in exercise had significantly higher serum aspartate aminotransferase and creatine kinase levels than rats fed low-protein diets and exercised. This means that while additional protein in the diet influences serum enzyme activity, further studies need to be done to assess how this increase in dietary protein affects the specific processes of muscle enzymes. (Note that prior exercise could influence the rate of increase in serum concentrations of enzymes after exercise independent of increases from greater intake of protein.[7])

How Much Protein?

As far back as 1840, the debate on how much protein a physically active person needs was in full swing. Researcher von Liebig in 1842[3,4,8] proposed that protein was the main nutrient for fuel for exercise; however, his idea was dismissed with the turn of the century as knowledge expanded about exercise metabolism and researchers discovered the roles of carbohydrate and fat in providing fuel during exercise. So, with almost a full century focusing on carbohydrate and fat, protein was left behind. Perhaps with the role of protein in the physically active out of sight and out of mind for the most part, the Recommended Daily Allowance for protein was (and still is) set at 0.8 g/kg body weight/day.[4] This value is based on data from mostly sedentary people; therefore, it does not account for the potentially greater needs of physically active people. Luckily for protein's sake, not all researchers pushed it aside. Lemon particularly took interest in examining protein in relation to physical activity and reported some interesting findings.[3–5,8]

It has already been established, from exploring how the body utilizes protein during endurance exercise, that as duration and intensity of physical activity increase so does the requirement for protein. Lemon proposed that the requirement for protein for endurance-training athletes be increased from the RDA of 0.8 g/kg body weight/day to 1.2–1.4 g/kg body weight/day,[3] while Meredith et al. found that the protein requirement in endurance-trained males averaged out to 1.26 g/kg body weight/day.[9] Furthermore, research from Burke et al. suggested that elite male endurance athletes may even need up to 1.5 g/kg body weight/day to satisfy their protein requirements,[10] and still other studies reported that moderate to high-intensity endurance exercise increases protein requirements to 1 g/kg body weight/day.[2] With all these proposed requirements, the American Dietetic Association revised its protein RDA in 1987, increasing it to 1 g/kg body weight/day for the physically active.[11]

Why all the discrepancies? The level of intensity, duration, point of exercise training, and possibly gender can all contribute to the varying need for protein for endurance athletes. Level of intensity as well as duration have already been addressed: the higher the intensity and longer the duration of exercise, the higher the requirement for protein (to a point). While increasing the protein requirement for endurance athletes is supported by research, benefits of protein intakes higher than 2 g/kg body weight/day have not been supported.[2] The stage of exercise training also factors into the protein requirement. Research supports that protein needs are higher for athletes in the beginning of their exercise program, and as the body trains longer and becomes adept at conserving protein, this need levels off.[11] Gender, too, appears to play a role in protein requirement. While exploring the nutritional needs of the female athlete, Manore concluded that the female endurance athlete has elevated protein needs in the range of 1.2–1.4 g/kg body weight/day.[12] However, both Tarnopolsky[11] and Lemon[3] reported research supporting that female endurance athletes may require a smaller protein increase than their male counterparts, since limited results find that women may utilize less protein during endurance exercise. Further studies on this matter need to be conducted.

The quality of the protein consumed, as discussed later, has the potential to affect its requirement. Few of the studies reviewed thoroughly accounted for the source(s) of protein that the endurance athletes consumed; therefore, this potentially contributes to the varying recommendations for the protein requirement.

Additionally, there are other reports stating positive effects of increased protein in the diet of endurance athletes. Researchers found that increasing protein intake at the start of an endurance exercise program reduced the development of anemia.[11] Also, further research found that increasing protein in the diets of female endurance athletes might reduce the occurrence of amenorrhea.[11]

Diet Composition and Its Effect on Protein Requirements

The composition of the diet has interesting effects on protein utilization and requirements. To begin with, total energy intake greatly influences the body's use of protein. When energy intake is excessive (promoting positive energy balance), protein is stored, whereas when energy intake is compromised (causing negative energy balance), degradation of body protein increases. This breakdown of body protein increases the body's overall need for protein.[2] Likewise, a demonstrated need for increased protein in the diet of an endurance athlete may be attributed to caloric deficiency and not necessarily a need for additional protein.[11]

When an endurance athlete consumes inadequate amounts of carbohydrate, this leads to rapid depletion of liver and muscle glycogen stores during endurance exercise. These depleted glycogen stores then lead to an increase in the utilization of protein by the body during exercise.[8] Exercise in conjunction with low-carbohydrate body stores stimulates BCKA dehydrogenase activity and promotes the breakdown of BCAAs to supply the liver with carbon skeletons for gluconeogenesis.[2] Important to understand, though, is that protein is likely to account for only 10 percent of total energy expenditure even when carbohydrate stores are low.[2] Thus, protein appears to serve an auxiliary role to carbohydrates, the main fuel source utilized during endurance exercise.

A study on the food intake and energy expenditure of participants during the Tour de France concluded that a high-protein intake might adversely affect carbohydrate intake (reduce it in some cases) and consequently reduce endurance. A diet insufficient in carbohydrates will lead to poor glycogen stores and a reduced energy supply for the endurance athlete's body to call upon during prolonged exercise.[13]

Clearly there needs to be a balance between carbohydrate and protein intake. While endurance exercise does appear to increase the athlete's need for protein, the athlete's need for carbohydrates should not be adversely affected by this increase in protein. For most of these studies concerning increased intakes of protein, the percentage of total calories from carbohydrates remained high, at around 55–65 percent, reinforcing the idea that carbohydrates are the most essential source of fuel during exercise, and protein is an auxiliary fuel source.

The Role of Protein in the Postexercise Diet

The role of postexercise protein consumption on protein metabolism is an interesting area of research.[14] One study exploring the value of protein in the postexercise meal found that consumption of a combined carbohydrate and protein meal after exercise increased the levels of the anabolic hormone insulin (which influences protein metabolism) higher than postexercise meals made up of only carbohydrates or only protein.[2] This result of increased insulin may be a consequence of the carbohydrate and protein meal having one-third more calories. Other research examining protein consumption after endurance exercise concluded that carbohydrate-protein mixtures increased levels of plasma insulin and growth hormone more than carbohydrates or protein alone.[2] These findings proposed that adding protein to carbohydrates for postexercise recovery may reduce breakdown of muscle and/or improve recovery. A possible reason for these findings is that since exercise promotes protein synthesis and oxidation of amino acids that lead to body protein breakdown and depletion of the amino acid pools, protein intake postexercise may spare muscle catabolism.[2] More research needs to be conducted in order to come to a final conclusion.

Where to Find Protein: Eggs?

Biological value (BV) is the gold standard for determining the quality of a protein. The higher quality the protein, the better source it is for our bodies. Why? The biological value of a protein is the extent to which the amino acid composition of the particular protein matches the amino acid composition of mammalian tissue.[15] Therefore, a protein with a high biological value is essential to an endurance athlete who oxidizes amino acids during exercise. The consumption of protein with high BV potentially supplies an athlete's body with enough essential and nonessential amino acids to fill the body's internal pools, which are continually drawn from to repair damaged muscles and oxidize amino acids during exercise. A diet of poor quality protein, lacking in some of the essential amino acids, will put the endurance athlete's body at risk of early fatigue and compromised performance. Remember that endurance exercise increases oxidation of the amino acid alanine in the muscle (proportional to exercise intensity), so consuming a protein source with adequate amounts of alanine, along with other complimentary amino acids, is essential for any endurance athlete desiring to perform optimally and ward off fatigue.

Eggs contain the highest quality of protein known; in fact, the egg is often the standard against which all other sources of protein are judged. The only superior source of protein is human milk because of the quantity of essential amino acids human milk supplies.[15] However, since human milk is not a readily available source, and because its acceptability as a protein source for post–breast-feeding age humans has not been evaluated, athletes do not consume it.

The RDA for protein is based on the assumption that the average mixed protein diet has a biological value of 70.[16] Therein lies the possibility that if an endurance athlete consumes a diet with an overall average biological value higher than 70, he or she may not need the additional protein that is recommended by current research. A diet composed of protein sources with a combined biological value higher than the biological value of 70 potentially provides an endurance athlete with the appropriate amounts of amino acids at a lower protein requirement than some of the proposed requirements. The egg has a biological value of 100.[16] This leads to the question of whether eggs as the main dietary source of protein would have potential benefits for an endurance athlete. This is still an area of speculation, and research needs to be done to determine if the amount of high-quality protein in the diet would affect the overall requirement for protein.

Eggs are an excellent source of the high-quality protein that an endurance athlete's body demands, but many athletes may restrict consumption of eggs due to the misconception that eating eggs causes increases in cholesterol. Although egg yolk is a concentrated source of cholesterol, studies show that intakes of one egg per day appear to have little or no effect on cholesterol levels and risk for coronary heart disease or stroke in healthy people.[17] Eggs do not need to be the sole source of dietary protein in an endurance athlete's diet, but consumption of eggs regularly along with a balanced diet of adequate energy and other high-quality protein sources has the potential to fuel an endurance athlete to perform at his or her best.

Are There Adverse Effects to Consuming More Protein?

While Lemon's research on protein requirements and athletes suggested that protein intake between 1.2 and 2 g/kg body weight/day does not cause problems in athletes,[17] excess protein and amino acid intake has been associated with adverse affects on renal function. Researchers Poortmans and Dellalieux studied whether these same adverse effects were apparent in healthy athletes who consumed a higher-protein diet than the current recommended RDA. The endurance athletes Poortmans and Dellalieux studied consumed 1.35 g protein/kg body weight (+/−0.12) daily. Findings showed no impairment of renal function based on the glomerular filtration rate and rate of calcium excretion on intakes up to 2.8 g/kg body weight/day in healthy athletes.[17]

Furthermore, Colombani et al. fed marathon runners a protein-supplemented drink (providing 1.8 g protein/kg body weight) during their race and found that the protein-and-carbohydrate–supplemented drink, compared with the control carbohydrate-only drink, did not affect myofibrillar protein breakdown as speculated, but importantly the added protein was proven to be absorbed and mostly oxidized with no apparent adverse effects on metabolism.[18] What this research revealed is that increasing the protein, to an extent, in the diets of endurance athletes has no apparent adverse metabolic effects. This along with Poortmans and Dellalieux's finding suggests that increasing protein intake in an endurance athlete's diet will not have adverse effects on either renal or metabolic function.

Conclusion

Our bodies need protein; there is no doubt about that. How much protein our bodies need is another question. The current RDA for protein is set at 0.8 g/kg body weight per day, but this is based on research of mostly sedentary people. A physically active person, especially an athlete participating in endurance activity, needs more protein than even the RDA for athletes of 1 g/kg body weight per day. Endurance activity causes muscle damage and oxidation of amino acids and stimulates protein synthesis. All these consequences of endurance activity lead to an increased need for protein to offset protein losses the body endures with the breakdown of body tissue and muscle. How much extra protein is needed is debatable and appears to depend upon point of training, intensity of training, diet composition, and gender. Recommendations, though, call for protein consumption in endurance athletes to be 1.2–1.5 g/kg body weight per day but not to exceed 2 g/kg body weight per day. The source of protein an athlete consumes should be of high biological value, making egg protein a potentially prime source of protein for athletes. Also, to fully benefit from increasing protein, athletes should not let protein intake interfere with total caloric intake or intake of carbohydrates. Finally, an increased amount of protein in a healthy athlete's diet has not been shown to have adverse effects on metabolism and/or renal function.

Increasing the protein requirement for endurance athletes is supported by significant evidence; however, further research needs to be conducted to explore how specific sources of protein affect this increased protein requirement. In theory, eggs, with their optimal biological value, appear to be the ultimate protein source for any serious athlete; therefore, further research is warranted of the effects of this high–biological value protein source on the protein metabolism and physical performance of endurance athletes.

References

1. Groff, J.L., and Gropper, S.S. Protein. In Advanced Nutrition and Human Metabolism. 3rd ed., Graham, L., ed. Belmont, CA: Wadsworth, 2000, pp. 163–215.
2. Rankin, J.W. Nutritional aspects of exercise—role of protein in exercise. Clin Sports Med 1999;18:499–511.
3. Lemon, P.W.R. Is increased dietary protein necessary or beneficial for individuals with a physically active lifestyle? Nutr Rev 1996;54:S169–S174.
4. Lemon, P.W.R. Do athletes need more dietary protein and amino acids? Int J Sports Nutr 1995;5:S39–S57.
5. Lemon, P.W.R. Dietary protein requirements in athletes. J Nutr Biochem 1996;8:52–60.
6. Kasperek, G.J., and Snider, R.D. Effect of exercise intensity and starvation on activation of branch-chain keto acid dehydrogenase by exercise. Am J Physiol 1987;252:E33–E37.
7. Hayward, R., Ferrington, D.A., Kochanowski, L.A., Miller, L.M., Jaworksky, G.M., and Schneider, C.M. Effects of dietary protein on enzyme activity following exercise-induced muscle injury. Med Sci Sport Exercise 1999;31:415–20.
8. Lemon, P.W.R. Effect of exercise on protein requirements. J Sports Sci 1991;9:53–70.
9. Meredith, C.N., Zackin, M.J., Frontera, W.R., and Evans, W.J. Dietary protein requirements and body protein metabolism in endurance-trained men. J Appl Physiol 1989;66:2850–56.
10. Burke, L.M., Gollan, R.A., and Read, R.S. Dietary intakes and food use of elite Australian male athletes. Int J Sports Nutr 1991;1:378–94.
11. McCarthy, P. How much protein do athletes really need? Phys Sportsmed 1989;17:170–75.
12. Manore, M.M. Nutritional needs of the female athlete. Clin Sport Med 1999;18:549–63.
13. Saris, W.H.M., van Erp-Baart, M.A., Brouns, F., Westerterp, K.R., and ten Hoor, F. Study on food intake and energy expenditure during extreme sustained exercise: the Tour de France. Int J Sports Med 1989;10:S26–S31.
14. Sizer, F., and Whitney, E. The proteins and amino acids. In Nutrition Concepts and Controversies, 7th ed., Bass, J., ed. Belmont, CA: West/Wadsworth, 1997, pp. 206–10.
15. Nutrient Values, USDA, September 9, 2000, http://www.rahul.net/cgi-bin/fatfree/usda.cgi.
16. Hu, F.B., Stampfer, M.J., Rimm, E.B., Manson, J.E., Ascherio, A., Colditz, G.A., Rosner, B.A., Spiegelman, D., Speizer, F.E., Sacks, F.M., Hennekens, C.H., and Willet, W.C. A prospective study of egg consumption and risk of cardiovascular disease in men and women. JAMA 1999;281:1387–94.
17. Poortmans, J.R., and Dellalieux, O. Do regular high protein diets have potential health risks on kidney function in athletes? Int J Sport Nutr Exercise Metab 2000;10:28–38.
18. Colombani, P.C., Kovacs, E., Frey-Rindova, P., Frey, W., Langhans, W., Arnold, M., and Wenk, C. Metabolic effects of a protein-supplemented carbohydrate drink in marathon runners. Int J Sports Nutr 1999;9:181-201.

Index

Page references in *italics* refer to tables or figures.

Abetalipoproteinemia, 143
Adenoviruses, 56
Aeroallergens, 171, 173
African Green monkeys, atherosclerosis studies in, 115
Age, effect on plasma lipoproteins, 90
Alanine, 186-187, 190
Albumen, 85, 159
 allergies to, 172
 coagulated, 4
 industrial, 6
Alcohol consumption, 89
Algae, green, for egg enrichment, 164
Algae, marine (golden), for egg enrichment, 40, 42, 125, 160, 165
Allergies, egg/food, 172
Alpha-Tocopherol, Beta-Carotene Cancer Prevention Study, 76
Alzheimer's disease, 15
 apo E and, 147-152
Amenorrhea, 188
American Dietary Guidelines, cholesterol, 166
American Heart Association
 Dietary Guidelines 2000, 79
 diet recommendations, 88-89
Americans, per capita egg consumption, 9
Amino acids, 185
 branch chain, 186
 essential, 83, 84
 oxidation of, 186-187, 190
Anemia, 188
 iron deficiency, 87
Animal feeding studies, cholesterol, 72-73
Animals, food, ω-3 fatty acids in, 124
Antibodies
 in allergic response, 171
 IgG, 61
 IgY, 61-*66*
 production in laying hens, 6
Antigens, 171, 172
Antioxidants
 and coronary disease, 15
 in diet, 93
 effect on COPs formation, 136
 in eggs, 90
 in poultry feed, 30
Apolipoprotein A, 103, 143
Apolipoprotein A-I, 95
Apolipoprotein B, 95, 103, 104, 143
 defective, 105-106
Apolipoprotein C, 143
Apolipoprotein C-III, 106
Apolipoprotein D, 143
Apolipoprotein E, 78, 104, 106
 biosynthesis, *146*
 function of, 143-144
 genes, 148-152
 health benefits of, 144-147
Apolipoprotein E-2, 148, 150-151
Apolipoprotein E-3, 148, 151
Apolipoprotein E-3-Leiden transgenic mice, 118
Apolipoprotein E-4, 149, 151
Apoproteins, function of, 144
Arachidonic acid, *23*, 38, 56, 57, 123
 in infant diets, 55
Arginine
 in apo E isoforms, 149-151
 supplementation, 151
Art, use of eggshells in, 6
Arteries, endothelial dysfunction in, 112
Arteriosclerosis, risk factors, 90
Aspartate aminotransferase, 187
Astaxanthin, 164
Asthma, 173
Atherogenesis
 animal studies, 72
 initiating, 112, *113*
Atherosclerosis
 animal models, 111-119

Atherosclerosis (*continued*)
  apo E-4 and, 149
  CETP and, 95
  and cholesterol, dietary, 111-112
  cholesterol-feeding studies, 72
  development of, 112-113
  nonhuman primate models, 114-116
  regression of, 116
  reversal of, 145
  risk factors, 89, 90, 92
  rodent models, 117-118
Athletes, protein requirements, 186-191
Atopic dermatitis, 173

Baboons, atherosclerosis studies in, 115-116
Barley, 159, 162
Basophils, 171
B-cells, 171
Beta-carotene, 49-50
Bile acids, 90, 91, 103
Biological value, proteins, 84, 189
Biotin, in eggs, 86
  cold storage and, 181
  thermal degradation of, 179-*180*
Birth defects, 15
Body fat distribution, 90, 92
Body mass index (BMI), 92
Body weight, excess, 92
Boiling, effect on egg nutrition, 178, 180, 182
Brain, developmental disorders, 125-127
Branch chain amino acids (BCAAs), 186
Branch chain α-keto acid (BCKA) dehydrogenase, 186, 189
Breast milk, 84
  DHA in, 127
  fatty acids in, 26-28

Calcium
  benefits of, 15
  in eggs, 10-*12*, 83, 86
Canadian Designer Eggs, 19
Cancer, 155
  colon, 15
  and ω-3 fatty acids, 21
Canola seed, 162
Canthaxanthin, 164
Capric acid, 111
Caproic acid, 111
Caprylic acid, 111
Carbohydrates, in diet, 187, 189
Cardiovascular disease. *See also* Coronary heart disease
  and egg consumption, 87-90, 93-97
  mortality rates, 127
  and ω-3 fatty acids, 21
  risk factors, 92-93
Carotenoids, in egg yolk, 164
Cebus monkeys, atherosclerosis studies in, 114
Cell cultures, hypoxic induction of, 63, 64, *66*
Centers for Disease Control, National Health and Nutrition Examination Surveys (NHANES), 9-10, 12, 14
Cephalin, in egg yolk, 56, *57*
Cereals, for poultry feed, 159, 162
CHD. *See* Coronary heart disease
Chick embryos
  and egg hypersensitivity, 172
  and vaccine production, 6
Chickens
  egg contents, *102*
  fat metabolism in, 46
Chocolate, 95
Cholesterol
  auto-oxidation of, 19, 31-32, 133-136
  in cell membranes, 134
  in eggs, 10-*12*, 56, 101
  excretion of, 90, 103
  metabolism of, 103-104
  negative perceptions, 20
  phobias, 20, 88
  redistribution of, 144, 145, 146, 147, 152
  synthesis and metabolism, 90-92
Cholesterol, dietary
  American Dietary Guidelines, 166
  and atherosclerosis, 111-112
  and coronary heart disease, 88, 104
    case-control studies, 74
    cross-sectional studies, 73-74
    independent effect, 77
    prospective studies, 74-77
  effect on serum/plasma cholesterol, 71, 87-88, 89-90, 93-97
  LDL:HDL ratio and, 78
  LDL-cholesterol and, 89
  recommended allowance, 101-102
  species variation in response to, 72
Cholesterol ester transfer protein (CETP), 95, 103
Cholesterol-feeding studies
  animals, 72-73
  human, 77-78
Cholesterol oxidation products (COPs), 133
  antioxidants and, 136
  and food, 135-136
  formation of, 134
  health risks associated with, 134
  serum, 135
Cholesterol, serum/plasma

  and cholesterol, dietary, 71, 87-88, 89-90, 93-97
  clinical studies, 77-78
  and coronary heart disease, 106-107
  dietary factors and, 105
  diets to reduce, 91-92
  egg-coronary heart disease relationship, 14-15, 104-105
    animal studies, 72-73
    individual responses, 105-106
  epidemiology, 73-77, 78
  LDL:HDL ratio, 78, 89
  lowering, 71
  and obesity, 92
  ω-3 fatty acid-enriched eggs and, 24, 42
Cholesteryl esters, 95, 103
Cholestyramine, 127
Chylomicrons, 103
Clolibrate, 127
Coagulation, of eggs, 4
Cocoa butter, atherogenicity of, 117
Coconut oil, 95, 162
  atherogenicity of, 117
Cognition, reduced, 15
Cold storage, eggs, 181
Colon cancer, 15
Conalbumin, 4
Continuing Survey of Food Intakes by Individuals (CSFII), 9-10, 12, *13*
Cooking, effect on egg nutrient content, 177-*181*
Copper
  cooking and bioavailability in eggs, 180-*181*
  egg white foaming and, 4-5
COPs. *See* Cholesterol oxidation products
Corn, 159
Corn gluten meal, 159
Corn oil, atherogenicity of, 117
Coronary artery calcification, apo E-4 and, 149
Coronary heart disease
  apo E and, 147-153
  cholesterol-associated risk of, 71, 78-79, 87, 88
  DHA and, 127-128
  diet and, 155
  egg consumption and, 14-15, 106
  egg-plasma cholesterol relationship
    animal studies, 72-73
    clinical studies, 78
    epidemiology, 73-77, 78
  hypercholesterolemia and, 106-107
  risk factors, 87
  spread of, 101
Coronary vascular disease, and egg consumption, 15
Cottonseed meal, 159
Cottonseed oil, 162
Creatine kinase, 187
Crustaceans, in laying hens diet, 165
CSFII, 9-10, 12, *13*
CVD. *See* Cardiovascular disease; Coronary vascular disease
Cyclin-dependent kinases, 128
Cyclins, 128
Cynomolgus monkeys, atherosclerosis studies in, 114
Cysteine, in apo E isoforms, 149-151
Cytokines, 58, *59*

Dairy products, 95
Death, causes of, 155
Dehydration
  COPs formation during, 135, 136, 137
  effect on egg nutrients, 182
Designer eggs, 22-23, 97-98
  cholesterol oxidation in, 31-32
  effect on plasma lipids, 24-26, 42
  mother's milk and, 26-27
  oxidative stability of, 29-32
  PUFA/SFA ratio, 20
  Vitamin E-enriched, 31, 46, 53
  yolk oil, 27-*28*
DHA. *See* Docosahexanoic acid
Diabetes
  antioxidant supplementation in, 93
  egg consumption and heart disease in, 94, 106
Diacylglycerol, 58
Dietary Guidelines 2000 (AHA), 79
Dietary Guidelines for American Adults, 93
Diets
  American
    average American diet (AAD), 91
    eggs in, 9-13
    fat content, 88-89
  antioxidants in, 93
  carbohydrates in, 187, 189
  Eskimo, 159
  fat-free, effect on apo E, *146*
  fiber in, 90
  hens, Vitamin E-enriched, 47
  high fat, 15, 91-92, 96
  infant, 55
  lipid-lowering, 96
  monounsaturated fatty acid rich, 96
  Paleolithic, 39
  postexercise, 189
  role of eggs in, 71
  saturated fatty acid rich, 89, 96
  vegetarian, 87

Diets (*continued*)
  weight control, 83
  Western, 96, 155
    ω-6:ω-3 fatty acids ratio, 37
Digestibility, egg proteins, 84
Docosahexanoic acid (DHA), *23*, 38, 42-43, 56, 57, 156
  -enriched eggs, 42, 97, 123-130
  food sources of, 125
  health benefits of, 123, 125-128
  in infant diets, 55
  in marine algae, 165
  recommended guidelines, 22, 23
Docosapentanoic acid (DPA), *23*, 128, 156
DPA. *See* Docosapentanoic acid
Duck eggs, contents, *102*

Eating habits, unhealthy, 94
Edison 300™ eggs, 125
Egg Beaters, 97
Egg consumption
  in American diets, 9-13
  atherosclerosis and, animal models, 118-119
  and cholesterol, 14-15
  decline in, 9, 20, *21*, 87, 141, 156
  and heart disease, 14-15, 74-77, 87-90, 93-97, 106
  limiting, 12-14
  and serum cholesterol, 104-105
Egg enrichment, products for, 159-166
Egg industry, response to cholesterol concerns, 20-21
Egglands Best, 97
Egg protein, 84
  effect of cooking on, 178
  storage and, 181
Eggs
  alternatives, 97
  antioxidants in, 90
  cholesterol content, 88, 101, 102-103
  composition of, 3
  cooking, 85-86
  decorative, 6
  dehydrated, 182
  DHA-enriched, 97
  digestibility, 84
  double-yolk, 85
  Edison 300™, 125
  enrichment diets for laying hens, 159-166
  fat in, 10-*12*, 84-85, 101-102
  flavor of, 5
  food uses, 3-5
  Greek, 40, *41*, 127
  hypersensitivity to, 172
  inedible, 6
  lutein-enriched, 97
  magic bullet effect, 141-152
  membrane protein, 6
  mineral content, 83, 85, 86
  modification of. *See* Designer eggs; Specialty eggs
  myths and misconceptions about, 87-97
  nonfood uses, 6-7
  nutritional value of, 3, 10-14, 45, 55, 83-84, 86-87, 156, *157*
  oils, 28, *29*
  ω-3 fatty acid-enriched, 22-32, 40-43, 46
  phobias, 88
  plasma cholesterol-coronary heart disease relationship
    animal studies, 72-73
    clinical studies, 78
    epidemiology, 73-77, 78
  powdered, 134, 136
  role in diet, 71
  selenium-enriched, 97
  storage of, effect of tocopherol on, 52-53
  substitutes, 104
  supermarket, 40, *41*
  as symbols, 6
  vitamin content of, 45, 53, 83, 85, 86
  vitamin E-enriched, 47-53, 97
Eggshells
  as calcium source, 3
  decoration of, 6
Eggstasy, 97
Egg white, 85
  coagulation of, 4
  foaming of, 4, 85
  inhibition of crystal formation, 5
  use in "fining" wines, 6-7
Egg yolk
  antibody, 61
  cholesterol content, 101, 102
  coagulation of, 4
  color of, 5
  composition of, 85-86
  emulsification of, 5
  modification of, 159
Eicosanoids, 58, *59*
  roles of, 38
Eicosapentanoic acid (EPA), *23*, 38, 42-43, 156
  recommended guidelines, 22, 23
Electrophoretic mobility shift assays (EMSAs), for anti-HIF-1 analysis, 62, 63
Embryos, chick, 6
Emulsification, of egg yolk, 5, 85
Endothelium, dysfunction of and lipoproteins, 112

Endurance exercise, protein need and, 186-191
Energy, from eggs, 10-*12*
EPA. *See* Eicosapentanoic acid
Eskimo diet, 159
Europe, meat consumption, 155-156
Exercise, protein need and, 186-191

Fat
  in eggs, 10-*12*, 84-85
  recommended allowance, 101-102
Fats, animal, atherogenicity of, 119
Fatty acids, effect on plasma LDL, 111
Fatty acids, essential, 123-124
  adequate intake (AI), 39, *40*, 42
  functions and pathways, 37-39
Fatty acids, monounsaturated, 156-157
  in eggs, 10
  and plasma cholesterol levels, 84
Fatty acids, n-3. *See* Omega-3 fatty acids
Fatty acids, omega-3. *See* Omega-3 fatty acids
Fatty acids, omega-6. *See* Omega-6 fatty acids
Fatty acids, polyunsaturated, 94-95, 156-157
  auto-oxidation of, 19
  in eggs, 10
  function of, 157
  interactions between, 123-124
  and plasma cholesterol levels, 84
Fatty acids, saturated, 73-74, 94-95
  atherogenicity of, 115
  and atherosclerosis, 111-112
  and cholesterol synthesis, 84
  in eggs, 10
  *trans*fatty acids, 73, 95
Feed, hen
  ω-3 fatty acid supplements, 40-42
  stability of, 29-31
  Vitamin E-enriched, 41
Feeding studies
  animal, 72-73
  human, 77-78
Fiber, and cholesterol excretion, 90, 147
Fining, use of egg whites in, 6-7
Fish, fatty acids in, 125, 156-157
Fish meal, 159, 161
Fish oils, 21, 22, 125
  cardio-protective effects, 159
  composition of, 157, *158*
  as feed supplement, 40, 42
  α-3 fatty acids in, 23, 38
Fish taint, 30, 164-165
Flaxseed, 38, 163
  as feed supplement, 40, 42
  lipid oxidation, 29-30
  for ω-3 PUFAs enrichment, 22, 23
  tocopherols in, 30-31
Foaming, egg, 4-5, 85
Folacin, in eggs, 86
Folate
  deficiency of, 15
  in eggs, 10-*12*
Folic acid, in eggs
  cold storage and, 181
  thermal degradation of, 179-*180*
Food disappearance data, 9
Foods
  allergies to, 172
  COPs in, 135-136
  dehydrated, 135, 136, 137
  fast/convenience, 88, 95
Formulas, infant, egg phospholipid-containing, 57-58
Framingham Heart Study, 74-76, 104
France, heart disease in, 15, 96
Free radicals
  α-tocopherol and, 53
  apo E isoforms and, 149, 150
  formation during egg drying, 134
  Vitamin E and, 46
Fruits, in diet, 77, 93

Gastrointestinal tract, and food allergens, 172
Gender
  effect on plasma lipoproteins, 90
  and protein requirements, 188
Genes, apo E, 148-152
Genetics, and risk of heart disease, 89
Glutathione, supplementation, 151-152
Gold Circle Farm Eggs, 97
Goose eggs, contents, *102*
Grains
  in diet, 77
  for poultry feed, 159
Greek eggs, 40, *41*, 127
Green algae, for egg enrichment, 164
Growth hormone, postexercise diet and, 189

Hamsters, atherosclerosis studies in, 117
Health Professionals Follow-up Study, 76, 93-94, 142
Heart disease. *See* Cardiovascular disease; Coronary heart disease
Heat, effect on egg protein, 4, 85-86
Hematococcus pluvialis, 164
Hens
  antibody production in, 6
  effect of age on egg cholesterol, 101
  egg enrichment diets, 159-166
  Vitamin E-enriched diet, 47

Heparin/manganese precipitin method, HDL measurement, 144
HIF-1. *See* Hypoxia-inducible factor-1
High-density lipoprotein:low-density lipoprotein ratio (HDL:LDL), effect of DHA on, 127-128
High-density lipoproteins (HDL)
  in feeding studies, 72-73
  ω-3 fatty acid-enriched eggs and, 24, 42
  particles, 144
  transfer of dietary cholesterol into, 103
HIV infection
  effect of egg phospholipid on, 58
  infants, 56
Homocysteine, serum/plasma, 15, 93
3-Hydroxy-3-methylglutaryl-coenzymeA (HMG-CoA), 103
3-Hydroxy-3-methylglutaryl-coenzymeA (HMG-CoA) reductase, effect of COPs on, 134
25-Hydroxycholesterol, 133, 134
Hypercholesterolemia, 92
  animal models, 118-119
  atherosclerosis and, 72, 73, 76, 112-113
  and coronary heart disease
    animal studies, 106
    human studies, 106-107
  familial, 105
Hyperlipidemia, 92
    apo E-4 and, 149
Hyperlipoproteinemia, 145, 149
Hyperresponders, 72, 105
Hypersensitivity, allergic, 171
Hypertension, 89, 92
Hyporesponders, 72, 105-106
Hypoxia-inducible factor-1 (HIF-1), production of IgY against, 61-*66*

ILP. *See* Intermediate-density lipoprotein
Immune system
  effect of egg phospholipid on, 58
  PUFAs and, 157
  sensitization of, 171
Immunoblots, for anti-HIF-1 analysis, 62, 63, 64, *65*
Immunofluorescence microscopy, for anti-HIF-1 analysis, 62, 63, *66*
Immunoglobulin A, secretory (sIgA), 172
Immunoglobulin E, 171, 172
    respiratory atopy and, 173-*175*, 173
Immunoglobulin G, 61
Immunoglobulins, in allergic response, 171
Immunoglobulin Y
  anti-HIF production, 61-*66*
  structure of, 61
Immunoregulation, mediators of, 58

Infants
  benefits of Designer Eggs, 26-27
  expected infections in, 56
  formulas for, 27
  nervous system of, 125-128
Inflammation
  chronic, apo E and, *146*
  mediators of, 58
  and ω-3 fatty acids, 21
  and plaque formation, 107
Inositol phospholipid, in egg yolk, 56
Institute for Health Realities, 152
Insulin
  postexercise diet and, 189
  PUFAs and, 157
Intermediate-density lipoprotein (ILP), 103
Iodine, in eggs, 86
  cooking and bioavailability, 180-*181*
Iron
  benefits of, 15
  in eggs, 10-*12*, 83, 86, 180-*181*
  and oxysterol formation, 135
Iron deficiency anemia, 87
Ischemic heart disease, 155

Japan
  dietary practices, 155
  heart disease in, 15, 96

α-Ketoisocaproic acid, 165
Keys, Ancel, 141

Lactate dehydrogenase, 187
Lactoovovegetarians, 83
Lard, 95
Lauric acid, 111
LCAT, 103, 143, 144
Learning ability, DHA and, 123, 126
Leather finishing, and egg albumen, 6
Lecithin, 85, 119
  in egg yolk, 56, *57*
Lecithin-cholesterol acyltransferase (LCAT), 103, 143, 144
Leucine, 165
Leukotrienes, 38, 58, *59*, 157
Lifestyle, sedentary, 89, 155
Light, effect on COPs formation, 134, 136
Linoleic acid, *23*, 37, 38, 123
  in egg yolk, 56
α-Linoleic acid (α-LA), in laying hens diet, 163-164
α-Linolenic acid (α-LNA), *23*, 38, 42-43, 123
  plant sources of, 160
  recommended guidelines, 22, 23
Linseed oil, 162

Lipid peroxidation products, 52-53, 135
Lipid Research Clinic
  Follow-up Study, 76
  Research Prevalence Study, 104
Lipids, food, 20-21
Lipids, plasma, effect of ω-3 fatty acid-enriched eggs on, 24, 42
Lipoprotein lipase, 103
Lipoproteins, in yolk, 160
Lipoproteins, high-density. *See* High-density lipoproteins
Lipoproteins, low-density. *See* Low-density lipoproteins
Lipoproteins, plasma, and risk of heart disease, 89-90
Lipoxins, 58
Liver, cholesterol synthesis in, 90-91, 103
Low-density lipoprotein:high-density lipoprotein (LDL:HDL) ratio, 78, 89
Low-density lipoprotein receptor (LDLR), 103-104
Low-density lipoprotein receptor-related protein (LRP), 103
Low-density lipoproteins (LDL)
  elevated, 87-88
  in feeding studies, 72-73
  ω-3 fatty acid-enriched eggs and, 24, 42
  oxidation of, 93
  receptors, 91
Lutein, 5
  benefits of, 15
  -enriched eggs, 42, 97
Lymphocytes, 171
Lysophosphatidylcholine, in egg yolk, 56
Lysophosphatidylethanolamine, in egg yolk, 56

Macular degeneration, age-related, 15
Magic bullet effect, apo E, 141-152
Magnesium, in eggs, 10-*12*, 86
Mahley, Robert, 144
Maize, 162
Major histocompatibility complex (MHC), 171
Malnutrition, 56
Manganese, in eggs, 86
Mannose-6-phosphate/insulin-like growth factor receptor (M6P/IGFII-R), 61
Margarines, 95
Marine oils. *See* Fish oils
Mast cells, 171
Meat consumption, 95, 155-156
Meat meal, 159
Meat-processing byproducts, for poultry feed, 160
Menhaden oil, in laying hen diets, 160-161
Mercury poisoning, apo E and, 147
Metals, heavy, apo E and, 147, 149, 150, 152
Methyl linoleate, atherogenicity of, 117
Methyl oleate, atherogenicity of, 117
Methyl stearate, atherogenicity of, 117
Mexico, CVD mortality rates, 15
MHC, 171
Mice, atherosclerosis studies in, 118
Microspheres, 164
Milk
  breast, 26-28, 84, 127
  whole, 95
Milo, 159
Minerals, in eggs, 83, 85, 86
  effect of cooking on, 180-*181*
Molasses, in poultry diets, 160
Monkeys, atherosclerosis studies in, 114-115
MUFAs. *See* Fatty acids, monounsaturated
Multiple Risk Factor Intervention Trial (MRFIT), 74, *75*
Muscle injury, exercise-induced, 186-187
Myocardial infarction, reducing risk of, 127-128
Myristic acid, 111

n-3 Fatty acids. *See* Omega-3 fatty acids
National Cholesterol Education Program (NCEP), 141
  dietary guidelines, 101-102
  Step I Diet, 96
  Step II Diet, 91
National Health and Nutrition Examination Surveys (NHANES), 9-10, 12, 14
National Health Organization, fat intake guidelines, *22*
National Institutes of Health, cholesterol workshop, 94
Necrotizing enterocolitis, 55, 56, 57
Nerve growth factor, 126
Nerve repair, apo E, 145
Nervous system
  effect of ω-3 fatty acids on, 125-127
  of infants, 125-128
Neurite elongation, 126
Neurodevelopment disorders, due to fatty acid deficiency, 125-127
Neurotransmitters, PUFAs and, 157
NHANES II, 89
NHANES III, 9-10, 12, 14, 74, *75*
Niacin, in eggs
  cold storage and, 181
  thermal degradation of, 179-*180*
Niacin, supplementation, 165

Nitric oxide (NO)
  apo E and, 149, 150-151
  formation during egg drying, 134
Nitrite, formation during egg drying, 134
NO, 134, 149, 150-151
Nurses' Health Study, 76, 92, 93-94, 142
Nutrient density, 83
Nutrition, eggs and, 86-87

Oats, 159, 162
Obesity, 89, 92
Off-flavors, in eggs, 5, 30
Oils, dietary, 47
  atherogenicity of, 117
Oils, vegetable, 39
Oleic acid, in egg yolk, 56, *57*
Olive oil diet, 91-92
Omega-3 fatty acid-enriched eggs
  fish taint in, 30, 40
  oxidative stability of, 29-32, 40-42
Omega-3 fatty acids, 19, 21-22, *23*
  benefits of, 21, 38-39, 42-43
  cardio-protective effects, 127-128
  CHD and, 20
  in food animals, 124
  human daily requirements, 53
  incorporation into yolk fat, 22-23
  metabolic pathway, *39*
  nervous system and, 125-127
  vision and, 123, 126-127
Omega-6:omega-3 fatty acid ratio, 157, 159
  designer eggs, 20
  dietary recommendations, 124
  in eggs, 20, 40
  enrichment diets and, 161, 166
  optimizing, 129-130
  Western diets, 37, 42
Omega-6 fatty acids, 19, 22, *23*
  metabolic pathway, *39*
Orotic acid, 165
Ovalbumin, allergies to, 172
Ovomucoid, allergies to, 172
Ovotransferrin, 4
  allergies to, 172
Oxidative stability
  ω-3 fatty acid-enriched eggs, 29-32, 40-42
  tocopherol-enriched eggs, 51
Oxygen homeostasis, HIF-1 regulation of, 62
Oxysterols, 133, 135

Palmitic acid, 111
Palm oil, atherogenicity of, 117
Pantothenic acid, in eggs
  cold storage and, 181
  thermal degradation of, 179-*180*
Parainfluenza viruses, 56
Pasta, COPs in, 134
Pasteurization, egg allergens and, 172
Peanut meal, 159
Peanut oil diet, 91-92
Peanut/peanut butter diet, 91-92
Pearl millet, 163
Phosphatidic acid, 58
Phosphatidylcholine, in egg yolk, 56
Phosphatidylethanolamine, in egg yolk, 56
Phospholipids, effect of ω-3 fatty acid-enriched eggs on, 24
Phospholipids, egg
  benefits of, 55
  components of, 56-57
  HIV-associated disease and, 58
  immune cells and, 58
  infant infections and, 57-58
  viral infectivity and, 58
Phosphorus, in eggs, 10-*12*, 86
  cooking and bioavailability, 180-*181*
Physical activity, protein need and, 186-187
Phytochemicals, 93
Plants, ω-3 fatty acids levels, 39
Plaque formation, 113-*113*
  and inflammation, 107
Plasmalogen, in egg yolk, 56
Platelet-activating factor, 58
Platelets
  effect of DHA on, 128
  PUFAs and, 157
Poaching, effect on egg nutrition, 178, 180, 182
Postexercise diet, 189
Potassium, in eggs, 10-*12*, 86
Poultry feed, 159-160
Poultry industry byproducts, in poultry feed, 159
Pregnenolone, 145
Progesterone, 145
Prostaglandins, 38, 58, *59*, 157
Prostacyclins, 38
Protein, animal, sources of, 155
Protein, dietary
  biological value of, 84, 189-190
  excess, 190-191
  metabolism of, 186-187
  need for, 185-186, 191
  recommendations, 187-188, 190, 191
  sources of, 188-190
Protein, egg, 4, 10-*12*, 84
Protein A, 61
Protein G, 61
PUFAs. *See* Fatty acids, polyunsaturated
Pyridoxine, in eggs, 86

cold storage and, 181
thermal degradation of, 179-*180*
Pyruvate, muscle, 186
Pyruvate kinase, 187

Rabbits, atherosclerosis studies in, 117
Radioallergosorbent test (RAST), 174
Rapeseed, 38
RAST, 174
Reactive oxygen species (ROS), 150
Remyelination, apo E and, 145
Renal function, and excess protein intake, 191
Resistance, specific/nonspecific, 171
Respiratory tract infections, 56
Retina, DHA in, 126, 129
Retinol, 182
Rhesus monkeys, atherosclerosis studies in, 114
Rhinitis, allergic, 173, 174
Rhinoviruses, 56
Riboflavin, in eggs, 10-*12*, 83, 86
cold storage and, 181
thermal degradation of, 179-*180*
ROS, 150
Royal Chemistry Society, 177, *178*, 179

Safflower oil, 162
Schizochytrium, 125
Scrambling, effect on egg nutrition, 178, 180, 182
Screenings, for poultry feed, 159
Seafood, fatty acids in, 156-157
Selenium
in eggs, cooking and bioavailability, 180-*181*
-enriched eggs, 42, 97
Seven Countries Study, 73-74, 141
SFAs. *See* Fatty acids, saturated
Shortenings, 95
Skin-prick tests, 174
Smoking, 89, 92
Smooth muscle, 150
Sodium, in eggs, 86
Soybean meal, 159, 161
Soybeans, 38
Spain, heart disease in, 15, 96
Specialty eggs. *See also* Designer eggs
ω-3 fatty acid-enriched, 40-43
Sphingomyelin, in egg yolk, 56
Stearic acid, 95, 111
Sterol biosynthesis, COPs inhibition of, 134
Storage
effect on COPs formation, 134, 136
effect on egg nutrient content, 181-182
Stress, 89, 155
Stroke, risk factors, 92
Sugar crystallization, inhibition of, 5
Sunflower seed, 163

Tankage, 159
Tau-protein, 150
T-cells, 171
Tetrabutylammonium (TBA)-reacting substances, 42
Thiamin(e), in eggs, 10-*12*, 83, 86
thermal degradation of, 179-*180*
Thiobarbituric acid (TBA), 51
Thiobarbituric acid (TBA)-reacting substances, 30
Thrombosis, arterial, 128
Thromboxanes, 38, 58, *59*, 157
effect of DHA on, 128
Thyroid function, apo E and, *146*
Tobacco smoke, 56
Tocopherol
antioxidant function of, 46
in chicken feed, 30-32
isomers of, 47-49, 50
α-Tocopherol, 47-49. *See also* Vitamin E
benefits of, 53
binding protein, 49
effect on COPs formation, 136
in laying hens diet, 163-164
all-rac-α-Tocopherol acetate, 49
dl-α-Tocopherol acetate, 47
δ-Tocopherol, 47-49
γ-Tocopherol, 47-49
Tocopherol enrichment, eggs
β-carotene and, 49-50
fatty acid composition and, 50
flavor and, 51-52
oxidative stability and, 51
storage and, 52-53
transfer efficiencies of isomers, 47-49
yolk fat and, 50
Triacylglycerols, 91
Triglycerides, serum, 103
effect of DHA on, 128
effect of ω-3 fatty acid-enriched eggs on, 24, 42
Turkey eggs, contents, *102*

United Kingdom, egg consumption, 156
United States, meat consumption, 155-156
Urticaria, 173
USDA Continuing Survey of Food Intakes by Individuals (CSFII), 9-10, 12, *13*

Vaccines
egg hypersensitivity and, 172
production in chick embryos, 6

Vascular smooth muscle, effect of ω-3 fatty acids on, 128
Vegetable oils
  atherogenicity of, 117, 119
  composition of, 157, *158*
  in laying hens diet, 161, 162
Vegetables, in diet, 77, 93
Vegetarian diet, 87
Vervet monkeys, atherosclerosis studies in, 115
Very-low-density lipoprotein (VLDL), 103, 144
Very-low-density lipoproteins, yolk-targeted (VLDLy), 160
Viruses, infectivity of, 58
Vision
  effect of DHA on, 123
  effect of ω-3 fatty acids on, 123, 126-127
Vitamin A, in eggs, 10-*12*, 45, 85, 86
Vitamin B_6, in eggs, 10-*12*
Vitamin B_{12}, in eggs, 10-*12*, 45, 83, 86
  cold storage and, 181
  thermal degradation of, 179-*180*
Vitamin C, supplementation, 142, 147
Vitamin D, in eggs, 45, 85, 86, 182
Vitamin E. *See also* α-Tocopherol
  effect on COPs formation, 136
  in eggs, 10-*12*, 85, 86
  -enriched eggs, 30, 41-42
  as feed supplement, 40, 42
  human daily requirements, 53
  for oxidation reduction, 164
  sources of, 46
Vitamins, B-complex, and coronary disease, 15
Vitamins, in eggs, 83, 85, 86
  effect of cold storage on, 181-182
  effect of cooking on, 179-*180*
Vitelogenins, in yolk, 160
VLDL. *See* Very low-density lipoprotein

Walnuts, 38
Weight loss, eggs and, 83
Western Electric Study, 77
Wheat, for poultry feed, 159
Women, Infants, and Children (WIC) program, 87
World Health Organization, ω-3 fatty acid recommendations, 124

Xanthophylls, 5

Yeasts, in poultry diets, 160
Yolk fat, 56-57
  function of, 50
  modification of, 22-23
  production of, 160

Zeaxanthin, 5, 15
Zinc, in eggs, 10-*12*, 83, 86
  cooking and bioavailability, 180-*181*